Good Blood

Good Blood

A doctor, a donor, and
the incredible breakthrough
that *saved* millions of babies

Julian Guthrie

ABRAMS PRESS, NEW YORK

Library of Congress Control Number: 2020932361

ISBN: 978-1-4197-4331-3
eISBN: 978-1-64700-015-8

Printed and bound in the United States
10 9 8 7 6 5 4 3 2 1

Abrams books are available at special discounts when purchased in quantity
for premiums and promotions as well as fundraising or educational use.
Special editions can also be created to specification. For details, contact
specialsales@abramsbooks.com or the address below.

Abrams Press® is a registered trademark of Harry N. Abrams, Inc.

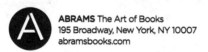

ABRAMS The Art of Books
195 Broadway, New York, NY 10007
abramsbooks.com

To all the brave and innovative doctors, nurses, donors, and volunteers on the front lines of medicine and research

CONTENTS

CHAPTER ONE
The Making of a Superhero

James Christopher Harrison peered out the paned living-room window of his family home in the railway town of Junee in New South Wales, Australia. He rubbed a circle where his breath fogged up the glass. His mates were out playing cricket in the street, and the ten-year-old pleaded with his mom to let him out.

"They don't have enough players!" he protested.

"Mum, they *need* me!" he tried again.

"They have a *terrible* bowler!" he said of the pitcher.

James's desperate entreaties went nowhere, blending into the background noise of the whistle of passing trains and the shouts and cheers of his friends in the street.

He had been ordered indoors until his latest cold passed, a torturous fate for a boy who just wanted to play like the rest of the kids in the small town. With big, dark brown eyes, light hair, and an innocent expression that masked a mischievous streak, James had always been a small and sickly child, picking up any cold or bug that went around Junee in the 1940s. During World War II, James's mom received extra rations of butter, milk, meat, and bread because of James's poor health. She tried her best to fatten him up with his favorites, bangers and mash and stone fruit pies.

Finally, after lunch, when the neighborhood boys had moved on from their game of cricket and taken their makeshift wicket with them, James resorted to a game of tag with his younger sister inside the house. No matter that he still hadn't finished his meal. As he raced around the house while eating, he ran into a wall, and the spoon in his mouth

1

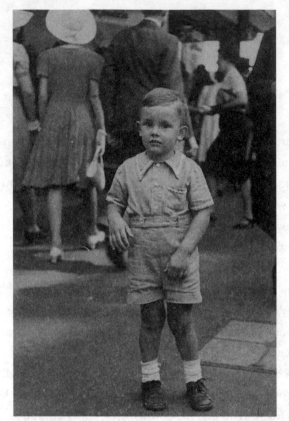

James Harrison at around age four, Junee, Australia.

was violently launched into the back of his throat. Off to the hospital they went—again.

When James wasn't battling some ailment, he was outdoors every moment he could grab, playing cricket or inventing battles, games, and races with his best friends, Ronny and Johnny Marshall.

One weekend afternoon, the three boys decided it was time for a race to the railroad tracks on their bikes. James had Ronny perched on the handlebars of his rickety bike, while Johnny was on his own bike, gunning to pass them. The boys had a block to go before crossing the train tracks that sliced through Junee. The whistle of the approaching train propelled them forward like the starter pistol at a race. James stood in his seat, gripped his handlebars, and glanced back at his competition.

"Holy smokes!" Johnny yelled.

Just then, a truck of some sort careened around the corner, coming out of nowhere. James veered but wasn't quick enough and smashed headlong into the back of the fast-moving vehicle. Johnny veered and just missed the pileup but slid across the road. Slowly, unsteadily, the bruised and battered boys picked themselves up.

"Crikey—what happened?" James said, helping Ronny up.

James scratched his head with a bleeding hand and said, "How did the medics get here so fast?"

"You idiot!" said one of the boys. "Look!"

When the reality of what had happened set in, the ribbing began: Only James Harrison would run into the back of an ambulance.

These were the kind of scrapes and scares that punctuated James Harrison's boyhood. But when he landed back in the hospital in 1951, it was for something far more serious than bruises, cuts, and bad colds. James, now fourteen, had caught something he couldn't shake. A bug had turned into bronchitis and then triple pneumonia. Penicillin was doing nothing to prevent the infection from spreading from one lung to the other. The tissue of James's lungs was inflamed, and he coughed constantly, complaining of sharp chest pains.

James was transported to St. Vincent's Hospital in Sydney in a bid to save his life. There, James's mom and dad, Peggy and Reginald, met with a young surgeon, Harry Windsor, who had honed his skills as a doctor during World War II, serving mostly in New Guinea with the Australian Army Medical Corps. Dr. Windsor had made a name for himself at St. Vincent's through his pioneering work in heart valve surgeries. He had established the thoracic surgery department, and even organized the hospital's staff cricket team, serving as coach. He endeared himself to his surgery patients by sleeping next to their beds.

But the operation involving young James would be Dr. Windsor's first pediatric pulmonary lobectomy, and James was in bad shape. The lobectomy of the lung was a surgical operation to remove an infected or diseased portion of the lung. Dr. Windsor was not certain whether the boy would make it.

"I've got my lucky penny," James told the doctor when they met, showing him a flattened coin. He explained that he and his friends would wait for the trains of Junee to get close before placing pennies on the tracks and watching them get squashed. The boys had pockets full of squashed pennies.

James charmed doctors and nurses alike with his chatter and good spirits. In the days leading up to the surgery, James endured relentless tests, gagging every time antiseptic was sprayed into his mouth, and closing his eyes when exploratory tubes were pushed down his throat. The tubes felt larger than his throat. When they were removed, James could finally uncurl his fists and run his fingers over his flat penny. The nurses came to him every day for blood draws. Of the four major blood groups—A, B, AB, and O—James was universal blood type O negative, the blood of choice in emergency rooms and for use in transfusions. Just 7 percent of the population has O negative blood. With no major blood group antigens, O negative blood is the ideal for recipients with any blood type. But James, as O negative, could only safely receive transfusions of O negative blood. The positive or negative factors on one's blood were determined by a protein called the Rh factor, which can be present (+) or absent (−), creating the eight most common blood types of A+, A−, B+, B−, O+, O−, AB+, AB−. Compatible blood for transfusions meant the difference between life and death.

The nurses complimented James on his prominent veins. He may have been weak and pale and prone to coughing bouts that were exhausting even to watch, but his veins were as strong as the Australian sun in summertime, he was told.

The nurses did their best to distract him from the tubes and needles by asking about girls, cricket, tennis, and school. James didn't mind having a gaggle of pretty nurses around, and he told them stories of how he earned pocket change by selling the eggs of his family's chickens to refugees who'd arrived in Junee after the war. He talked gaily about his mishaps and adventures, including the time he'd scared his mother nearly to death by flinging himself across the train tracks to see whether an approaching train would stop. His mates Ronny and Johnny had pulled him off the tracks in the nick of time. Peggy, upon learning of the incident, said she'd kill him herself and chased after him with a wooden spoon.

The nurses and nuns at St. Vincent's were briefed on the risks of James's surgery. They admired how James did a lot with a little, and could only imagine what sort of mischief he'd get into if given the gift of good health.

When surgery day arrived, James's parents forced reassuring smiles while fighting back tears. James's father, Reginald, was a mechanic who fixed the wheels on the country's steam-powered locomotives. He never missed a Sunday church service, sang in the choir—becoming emotional with every rendition of "Amazing Grace"—and was the town Santa Claus. As Dr. Windsor explained the surgery, Reginald nodded, solemn and deferential. Dr. Windsor had told the Harrisons that he believed the best hope for their son was to remove the necrotic and infected parts of his right lung before it spread to the left side. There was a chance the doctor would have to remove the entire right lung. James's single remaining lung could inflate to take up some of the extra space, the doctor explained, allowing him—assuming all went well during surgery—to function normally. But the high-risk surgery would culminate in a high-risk recovery. Lung surgery involved a great deal of bleeding. Patients who bleed excessively during surgery are at risk of continuing to bleed after surgery, because the loss of platelets impairs the body's ability to make clots.

James's younger sister, Margaret, who was nine years old, stood next to their mother. She knew the situation was serious because they were in the big hospital in Sydney, rather than in their small hospital in Junee. A Sisters of Charity nun walked beside the gurney that carried James. The nun told Peggy and Margaret that she would stay with James through the operation. For the first time since being hospitalized, James was scared. His long bouts of coughing had left him depleted. He'd had a fever off and on and had been in the hospital for a week now. He just wanted to get back to racing around town and playing cricket in the street. But he smiled bravely. He could see his parents were worried. A few minutes later, it was time for him to be wheeled away.

In the operating theater, an overhead light the size of a manhole shone on James. Faces in white cloth masks peered down at him; he recognized the nurses by their eyes. The anesthetist, inducing with ethyl chloride spray on a cloth, and continuing with an ether drip, told him to count back from ten. Instead, James launched into one of his sweet but rambling tales. "My schoolmates like to sneak a puff of a ciggy behind a building where the teachers can't see," he began. "I never once did that . . ." James trailed off as the anesthesia took hold. The team quickly went to work, double checking the inventory on tables and trays, including the sponges, towels, clamps, scissors, scalpels, saws, and other instruments. A glass bottle of blood hung on an IV stand next to James. The use of glass bottles for blood donations, surgery, and storage dated to World War I—then the first glass cylinders were coated with a film of paraffin to delay clotting, and packed into ammunition boxes converted into shipping containers filled with ice and sawdust.

Dr. Windsor conferred with the anesthetist and checked James's vital signs. He made the first incision below James's sternum. He slowly cut in what he called a "lazy S" pattern toward the wall of the shoulder blade and spine. He cut through skin first, then fat—James was thin as a rail—and then continued the incision into the subcutaneous tissue and muscle. When he reached the chest wall and the rib cage, a nurse handed him a rib spreader. Dr. Windsor began to spread James's ribs, one crank at a time, like jacking up a car to repair a tire. To get to the muscles between the ribs and access the lungs, he would need to remove at least one rib.

Reaching the lungs, Dr. Windsor could see that the infection was worse than he had thought. The three lobes of James's right lung appeared necrotic. The tissue had died, and the space between the lung and the chest wall was filled with abnormal fluid, bacteria, and pus. Dr. Windsor suctioned the infection and peeled away hardened areas, like he was removing skin from an orange.

Sweat formed on Dr. Windsor's brow. James's blood pressure was dropping; he was hemorrhaging.

"More blood!" Dr. Windsor ordered. He had never had a patient undergo such a massive transfusion. The use of transfusions had developed over several centuries, beginning with the discovery of the circulation of blood in 1628 and the first recorded successful blood transfusion in England in 1665, when a dog was kept alive by the transfused blood of other dogs. Further advancements had been made during World War II. The understanding of blood type compatibility involving the Rhesus factor—giving people the positive or negative to their blood type—was just over a decade old.

James had about eight pints of blood in his body and was losing blood as fast as it was being replaced. He had already received four pints of transfused blood—half the volume of the blood in his body. James's breathing grew shallow and rapid and his heart rate accelerated.

More bottles of blood were rushed in for transfusion. Dr. Windsor, focused on the surgery, was relying on his nursing team to ensure that blood typing and crossmatching were executed to exclude incompatible mixtures for transfusion. A nurse wiped the doctor's brow. Others sopped up the blood around the incisions. Towels heavy with blood were piled on trays. Dr. Windsor eyeballed the amount of blood he had suctioned from James and released into canisters. James's arteries were constricting to prevent more blood loss, which could lead to organ failure. In the corner, the nun prayed the Rosary, her fingers moving from one bead to the next. The hours passed with this dance between life and death. Death approached, death was averted. Blood was lost, blood was given.

In the waiting room, James's family grew more anxious as day turned into night. Ten hours into the surgery, Reginald and Peggy still knew nothing. They tried not to imagine the worst.

Finally, after eleven hours of surgery, Dr. Windsor was done. James had received thirteen units of blood. His blood was no longer his own.

The necrotic lung tissue was on a tray. Dr. Windsor sewed up James's lungs, then the tissues, progressing methodically as if closing a door to each room he had entered. He then focused on closing James up. He sutured James's skin, making more than one hundred stitches by hand in a jagged line running from his chest to the middle of his back. As he worked, more transfused blood flowed into James's veins, moving through his wan body, replenishing what he'd lost. Now this brave boy, a fighter if ever there was one, would need to get through recovery.

When James awoke in the ICU, his family was all around him. The nun was there, too; she had stayed with him through it all. James faced tough days ahead, and he would have to remain in the hospital for months. He looked around his room. His parents were beaming, and told him he had done great. His father came bedside and clasped his hand.

"You were saved by the blood of strangers," Reginald said. "You would have died without the gift of blood."

James knew that his father was a regular blood donor. With a sense of responsibility that belied his daredevil acts on the train tracks, James told his family, "I will return the favor."

No one could have known that day in 1951 how true that was. The transfused blood that saved his life was altering James's very chemistry, mobilizing his antibodies, changing him at a molecular level—and creating a life force for others.

CHAPTER TWO
The Blood Detective

Hundreds of passengers cheered and waved from the deck of the *Queen Mary* as the impressive ocean liner entered New York harbor in the summer of 1955. The spectacular Manhattan skyline and the nearby Statue of Liberty captivated émigrés and tourists alike, and everyone on board wanted to cherish the moment of the ship's berthing at Pier 90, their gateway into the United States.

But one passenger was curiously absent among the celebrating masses. Three decks below, twenty-four-year-old John "Doc" Gorman was stealing one last glimpse of a thing of beauty: the engine room, with its massive turning gears, propellers, pipes, turbines, and valves that adjusted the amount of steam that powered the ship. For Gorman, a young doctor traveling on a cheap fare from Australia to make his name in America, the luxurious splendor of the *Queen Mary's* ballrooms paled in comparison to the engine room, even with its extreme heat and excessive noise.

"Look at that," Gorman said to himself while studying the machinery and scribbling notes. During his voyage, he had learned the intricacies and force of the engines, which produced sixteen tons of steam heated to 700 degrees Fahrenheit (370°C) every minute. From his perspective, the other passengers didn't know what they were missing. He had been thrilled early in the voyage when some of the machinists invited him in for a tour. Maybe they took pity on him, seeing that his cabin was next door to the engine room.

Gorman bid farewell to the greasers, firemen, engineers, and trimmers in the engine room, grabbed his bag, and dashed through the narrow passageways and up the flights of stairs. They had arrived in America! On the main deck, out of breath, he beheld another glorious sight—the Empire State Building, the tallest manmade structure on Earth.

Gorman had never seen a skyscraper, let alone a whole city of skyscrapers. New York City had been his dream destination for as long as he could remember. It was big, fast, tall, and bustling—a place of ideas. He had been a big fish in a little pond back home in Australia. Now he wondered whether he could become a big fish in this place teeming with the ambition and industry of nearly eight million people.

What Gorman knew of America came from copies of the *New Yorker*, *Newsweek*, and *Time* that his father shared with him at home in Bendigo, the town where gold was discovered in Australia. As a boy, he read the magazines cover to cover in his dusty workshop in the family's garage, where he toiled away on circuits, built boomerangs, and pieced together radios from vacuum tubes. Growing up, he'd wanted to be an engineer or physicist, and he was also drawn to math, regularly challenging himself to feats of mental arithmetic, from predictive modeling to concepts of integrals and derivatives and more. His father was his best teacher.

By the age of five, John knew the names of every country and every capital in the world. He did advanced math while still in elementary school.

As the first-born son of two doctors, it was expected that young John would also become a doctor. He started medical school at sixteen, having skipped grades because of his high test-scores—something that confounded those who knew him to sleep through classes or miss them altogether. John wasn't a fan of waking early or taking orders. For as long as he could remember, he had found school tedious and looked for any opportunity to play hooky. One day when he was around seven years old, he ditched school to head to town. Turning the corner, he ran

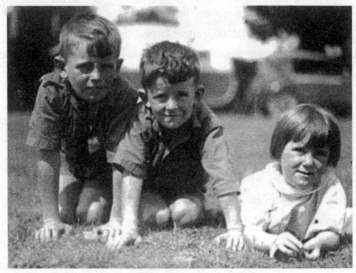

Left to right: John Gorman with his younger brother, Frank,
and sister Jocelyn, Rochester, Australia.

smack into his father, who was more than a little surprised to see his boy cruising down Main Street in the middle of a school day. During his six years of medical school at the University of Melbourne, his friends—who christened him "Doc" before he was one—also marveled at how he passed his exams when he seemed to always be sleeping, inventing, or golfing.

Now navigating the busy streets of Manhattan, Gorman was unlikely to run into anyone remotely familiar. But the sheer rush of so many people was its own kind of jolt. After taking several wrong turns and stopping to crane his neck at the skyscrapers, he finally arrived at his studio apartment. He had free room and board and would earn $50 a month as a pediatrics resident at St. Francis Hospital in the South Bronx. Settling into his new home, he began to unpack his few belongings, including a treasured book, *Ideas Have Consequences*, given to him by his father. He found the book interesting, but it was the title that spoke to him.

With the nearly two-month journey behind him, John's thoughts returned to the morning he'd left Australia. He'd sailed out of the port of Melbourne on a ship called the SS *Orcades*. There he stood on the top deck, squeezed shoulder to shoulder with other passengers, everyone holding streamers connected to loved ones on the dock below. John was connected to his mother, Doris, by a white streamer that seemed to run the length of a football field. John held one end, Doris the other. As the ship's horns sounded and the *Orcades* slowly pulled away, streamers broke all around, floating through the air like confetti. John and his mother held theirs for as long as possible, with John stretching out beyond the deck's rail and his mother moving toward him on the dock below. But in an instant, the tie between mother and son broke. Doris waved tearfully, still holding her part of the streamer. The image played over and over in his mind. He was now on his own. He would focus on his work—and on becoming someone of note.

Drifting off to sleep in his new apartment, John remembered the stories of his forebears. Arduous journeys had marked the start of new lives in Australia for both sides of his family. His grandmother Aggie Maguire was nineteen years old when she traveled from England to Australia in 1888 with her older sister and brother. Her brother died along the way. By the time Aggie was thirty-nine, she had nine children and was a widow, forced to adapt to each new challenge. Similarly, the first Gormans to leave Ireland arrived in Australia in 1839 as indentured laborers or "bounty immigrants" aboard the fully rigged sailing vessel the *William Metcalfe*. They spent months at sea, cramped into shared living quarters where disease and infection spread rapidly. Those who died were wrapped in canvas and tossed overboard. The Gorman clan had a history of quick-minded adaptations.

It didn't take John Gorman long in his pediatrics residency to discover important things about himself and the practice of medicine. He was surprised and dismayed to find that mothers in America challenged just about every diagnosis and recommendation he made. Exasperated, he told another resident: "In Australia, patients listen to every word you say. The doctors are king. Here, it appears that mothers run the case. I suggest antibiotics. They suggest no antibiotics." No matter how firm he was in his diagnoses, families of patients were either skeptical or opposed and relentless in their questions.

What he didn't admit was that he was terribly shy and not at all fond of interacting with people. He didn't mind practicing medicine, but he would prefer to do it without the patients. It had been the same in childhood, where it was always his younger brother, Frank, who was the gregarious one. The two boys had had different interests from the start. Where John loved the challenges of math, geography, and tinkering in his workshop, Frank was interested in sports and had a spectacular imagination. John had watched his brother with envy. Frank had a way with people, and a way of turning mundane things into fun and elaborate games, taking small toy trucks and developing games that everyone wanted to play. Frank had always been outgoing and had a lot of friends; John was the reclusive one.

Gorman soon maneuvered his way out of pediatrics at St. Francis and into a new job at the prestigious Columbia Presbyterian Hospital in Manhattan. Columbia had started a new residency program in clinical pathology and laboratory medicine. Gorman cycled through microbiology, hematology, and chemistry before finding his calling in blood banking and laboratory medicine.

The pathology lab was his new workshop. It was quiet, full of instruments, and devoid of patients—perfect for the taciturn tinkerer. He could arrive at work mid-morning and had weekends to himself. Already he had started working on a machine that would automatically perform one of the more tedious of the routine blood tests, the prothrombin time test, which measures the amount of clotting factor in a patient's blood.

Columbia had opened one of the first blood banks in the world, and Gorman was the teaching hospital's very first clinical pathology resident. The blood bank had an impressive history, beginning with Charles Drew, who in 1938 received a Rockefeller fellowship to study at Columbia and train at Presbyterian Hospital. Drew went on to develop a method for processing plasma—the blood component that delivers nutrients, proteins, and hormones around the body—and preserving and drying it to be reconstituted when needed. As World War II escalated in Europe, Drew was asked to lead a medical effort known as Blood for Britain, in which he organized the collection of blood plasma from New York hospitals to be shipped out to treat casualties of the war. Drew, who was black, would later withdraw as head of the American Red Cross because of the military's order to segregate blood by race, with blood donated by "Negroes" to be used only for other "Negroes."

Gorman was thrilled to have landed in a place with an impressive pedigree and was energized by the enthusiasm of researchers around him. It felt like great science was done there. Pathology was the basis of medicine and Gorman's road to understanding disease. He knew he could move from blood banking to immunology, which he found fascinating, and into the biochemistry of cells. Columbia was a place where there was pressure to get published, win the big prizes, and grab headlines.

Outside of work, Gorman, who had light blue eyes and a thatch of dark hair, began to socialize with a small group of colleagues and nurses. Together they'd head out for dinner or take in a Broadway show. Gorman loved big American cars, and had bought a pale green Ford, about the size of his studio apartment. One night out on the town, Gorman drove to dinner as the doctors and nurses swapped stories. Out of the blue, a nurse in the back decided to extend her legs all the way out the window. Her timing was impeccable: The police were cruising by. Lights flared, sirens sounded, and Gorman was pulled over, taken to the station, and tossed into a holding cell with a motley mix of drunkards and criminals. Clad in his usual attire of wool trousers and a white button-down shirt and tie under a rumpled V-neck sweater, Gorman declared repeatedly to no avail that he was a doctor at Columbia. Finally, at around three A.M., a friend arrived and had him sprung. On the way home, Gorman kept asking, "Why would the girl do that?"

On another occasion, Gorman was invited to a five-story, red brick townhome on the Upper East Side. As he sat in the sunlit family room, which opened to a lovely garden, in walked a gorgeous blonde, maybe twenty years old. She plopped down on the sofa next to Gorman and beguiled him with her charm. *This is my lucky day*, he thought. He was sure she was keen on him. But just as he was about to ask for her number, in walked a young man—her boyfriend. He hadn't even had time to learn her name. Afterward, Gorman's friends laughed at the story, saying, "That's Henry Fonda's daughter—we were at his house. His daughter is Jane. Jane Fonda."

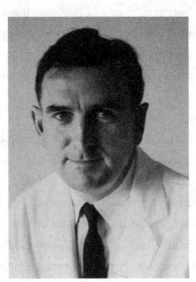

John Gorman as a resident at Columbia Presbyterian Hospital in New York, 1959.

Gorman found safer ground back in the quiet of his lab at Columbia. There, he worked on a range of projects, from rethinking lab equipment to readying blood for transfusions. Mistakes happened more than anyone would like to admit. As he saw it, blood banks had three main problems: incompatible transfusions, where the patient was given the wrong blood, something that could bring a range of reactions, from inflammation to sudden death; hepatitis, which was being transmitted though donated blood; and Rh disease, which was taking the lives of tens of thousands of fetuses and newborns each year, wreaking havoc on families around the world. Blood bankers and researchers across the globe were struggling to understand and treat this blood-based disease.

There was no test for hepatitis—a rugged virus that plagued blood banks—and no cure for Rh disease. Though it had only been named and diagnosed for two decades, the symptoms of Rh disease had been recorded as early as 400 BCE. Some in the medical community speculated about famous cases of the blood disease—long before the Rh factor was discovered and named. King Henry VIII and the first two of his six wives, Catherine of Aragon and Anne Boleyn, had multiple miscarriages and stillbirths. In keeping with the mechanism of Rh disease, which typically spares the first child but is more destructive with each subsequent pregnancy, Catherine of Aragon had a healthy first child, Mary, and then suffered multiple miscarriages.

Gorman was in his office one day in the fall of 1959 working on ideas for a "lock" that would ensure safer blood transfusions, when in bounded a strongly built doctor who energetically extended his hand.

"Vince Freda, researcher and doctor," the man said, shaking Gorman's hand. Dr. Freda, who had a crew cut and thick black-rimmed glasses, was close to Gorman in age, and had gotten his medical degree at New York University.

Gorman, who had heard of Vince Freda but hadn't met him, introduced himself as a pathology resident from Australia. The men exchanged pleasantries and Gorman invited him to have a seat. Freda, it turned out, was a former air force flight surgeon who had studied for a year under Alexander Wiener, a protégé of none other than Karl Landsteiner, "the Father of Blood Science."

Landsteiner, the world's leading blood researcher, had won the Nobel Prize in 1930 for his work in the discovery and classification of the blood of humans into the A, B, AB, and O groups. The classifications refer to antigens—the substances which produce antibodies—on the surface of red blood cells. In 1937, Landsteiner and Wiener, working at the Rockefeller Institute for Medical Research in New York, had discovered the Rh antigen—85 percent of people have the protein on their red cells, and are thus positive, while only 15 percent lack it, and are negative. Weiner called it the Rh factor, naming it after the Rhesus monkeys used as test subjects.

Gorman was full of questions and eager to hear stories about Wiener and Landsteiner.

Freda was as warm and gregarious as anyone he'd met, readily sharing stories and applauding the work of others. Freda talked about Wiener's development of a complete blood exchange transfusion in a newborn with Rh disease, a treatment that led to a significant decline in the infant mortality rate. The procedure required him to replace the Rh-positive blood of the infant with Rh-negative blood. Wiener taught Freda how to perform these transfusions.

Wiener had told Freda that the discovery of the Rh factor was no accident, but the result of Landsteiner's earlier work on the nature of antigens and antibodies. While Wiener and Landsteiner didn't immediately understand its significance—new antigens were being discovered all the time—Wiener soon realized that the Rh factor was associated with problems in transfusions. His research showed that although someone with Rh negative blood would typically be unharmed the first time he received an Rh-positive blood transfusion, the transfusion would prompt the recipient to create antibodies that would make a second such transfusion dangerous or even deadly. The discovery of the Rh factor made possible the safer use of blood for transfusions.

At the same time Wiener and Landsteiner were working in New York, another researcher, Philip Levine, also a protégé of Landsteiner, was zeroing in on the mechanism of Rh disease. Where Wiener had identified the Rh factor and its risk to transfusion patients, Levine, working from his lab in New Jersey, was looking at how the Rh factor harmed babies.

Gorman liked Freda immediately, and found his knowledge impressive and optimism contagious. But soon, he watched as Freda sank lower in his chair and began to rub his brow. He exhaled loudly, looking exhausted.

Gorman asked whether he was okay.

Freda shook his head, telling him that he had just lost another baby.

"It's this Rh disease," Freda said, "this incompatibility between baby and mother that is killing babies." Gorman nodded. He had studied Rh disease in medical school and knew the problem occurred when a baby inherited Rh positive blood from the father, and the mom's blood was Rh negative. The mother's antibodies, made by the immune system to fight things it didn't want in the body, destroyed the baby's red blood cells, causing anemia, miscarriages, and death in the baby. No one knew how to stop it, and thousands of babies were affected in the United States alone each year.

Gorman told Freda about his days as a medical student in Melbourne. During his obstetrics rounds, all students were required to sleep in the hospital. When the bell rang at three A.M., he and the other students knew to quickly dress and rush down to emergency. In this case, they had been summoned to watch a surgery involving a baby who was suffering from Rh disease. Gorman told Freda he remembered watching the doctors perform an exchange transfusion by using a needle to slowly remove some of the baby's blood and replace it with donated blood. The procedure lasted for hours, but it ended with the baby dying on the operating table.

Freda listened intently. As an ob/gyn, Freda was the one who had to tell mothers and fathers that their babies hadn't made it, and explain that the problem was rooted in something as simple—yet mysterious—as one's blood group. Freda told Gorman that he had lost too many babies to this blood disease: babies who died in utero; babies who arrived in the world yellow from jaundice; and babies with severe Buddha-like abdominal swelling, and permanent brain damage. Some newborns waged a heroic fight, surviving for days or even weeks. One baby died after undergoing dozens of transfusions. Freda saw how the losses wrecked parents and left the mothers with a sadness that never went away.

Gorman could see that this was Freda's mission He told Freda that he had done autopsies on Rh babies who had come into the world stillborn, brain damaged, or with little chance of surviving. This was one of the more difficult things to see in his residency.

Freda nodded with understanding. He enjoyed talking with this young Aussie and found him to be a keen listener brimming with ideas and energy. The kinship between the two was instant, and they talked nonstop, until Freda was pulled away.

Before leaving, Freda paused and said, "Rh is a disaster. We need to figure out how to stop this disease."

Gorman saw the determination on Freda's face.

"We do," Gorman nodded. "Agreed."

Gorman had always been drawn to simple inventions for complex problems. And Freda had come to the disease through the very men who discovered it.

Freda, now halfway out the door, had an idea.

"I need every file that you have on mothers who have been treated for this disease and who have had problems with their pregnancies."

Gorman understood. He had already begun to zero in on blood and an unresolved problem of immunology: how the body detects and identifies an antigen and produces a specific antibody that will selectively search and destroy it. The unsolved questions of Rh disease were clear: Why would a mother's body defy an almost universal law of nature and wage an attack against her own unborn child? How could this be stopped?

Gorman watched Freda head down the hallway before turning to head back into the lab.

He quickly called in a technician. He would need help pulling together every file on every woman treated at Columbia for Rh disease. On that day, Gorman—with Freda as his partner—committed to becoming a detective in the vexing global scourge of Rh disease. Gorman had been enthralled with the study of blood from his early days in medical school. The right blood could save your life, but the wrong blood type could end it. It was bright in the arteries, duller in the veins. Blood was life and death, health and disease. It delivered oxygen, and it could stop your breathing. Blood abounded in contradictions. It was given for free but was a commodity more precious than gold. It was powerful, sacred, and feared. Made in the bones, blood was always dying, always renewing.

In short order, Gorman had hundreds of 3x5 cards that had been created by residents who came before him and stored in a tall metal cabinet. The small yellow cards, spread across the tables in the blood lab, were a puzzle that needed to be pieced together.

Behind the numbers, names, and shorthand notes on the cards were lives altered: dreams of families dashed; nurseries decorated but never used; siblings that never made it home; baby names chosen and laid to rest. The cards in this one lab alone could stretch from wall to wall. Columbia Presbyterian was just one hospital in one city in one state. The same losses existed everywhere, from New York to Australia, from wealthy countries to the developing world. Gorman didn't have to turn to complex math formulas or predictive analysis to know that the losses of past and present carried into the future: Countless descendants would never have a chance. Saving one baby could preserve a generation.

This global blood disorder between mother and child was a ghost that had already been chased for decades. But no one was any closer to catching that deadly apparition and halting its path of destruction. Gorman, whose mind raced far ahead of his teachings, joined in the chase of the rare and elusive: to know something no one had ever known. But he understood, in talking with Freda, that this was bigger than any prize. Each 3x5 card before him represented a life.

CHAPTER THREE
A Home at the Bank

James Harrison plopped down in a chair in the Sydney blood bank and extended his legs. He had to laugh—his feet were sticking out the window toward the bustling streets below. "Surely a sight for passersby," he said to a nurse, who was preparing to draw blood from the crook of his right arm. The donor room at the Red Cross blood center could accommodate two people but was big enough for just one recliner. So, with the other chair occupied, James had assumed the position—legs extended out the window.

"This won't hurt a bit," the nurse said reassuringly. Yet James, despite having donated blood for almost three years now, averted his eyes. He could never watch the needle enter his skin.

James was no longer a sickly, accident-prone kid who raced around Junee on his rickety bike. He was approaching his twenty-first birthday, was strongly built, and stood six feet two. He had grown into a good-looking young man with bright dark eyes, and a smile his mother said would melt the ladies' hearts.

The perilous surgery in 1951 to remove his infected lung had done more than save James's life. It had given him a new life. After two months of recovery in St. Vincent's Hospital—with insistent nurses escorting him on walks up and down the hallways—he emerged healthy and stayed that way. He rarely caught so much as a cold. It was as if his immune system had been supercharged. James's father, a fan of comic books, spun stories of how his son had received transformative blood, like Peter Parker, who becomes endowed with spider powers after being bitten by a spider, or the Flash, who gets super speed when

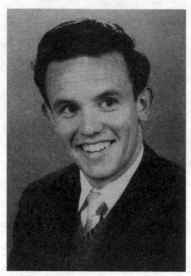

James Harrison at around age twenty, Sydney, Australia.

lightning strikes his lab and he is doused with chemicals. With his new powers, James no longer had to sit idly by in his house, waiting for his mother's permission to go outside. Instead, he played cricket in the streets, tennis all summer, and rugby through the winter. He became the athlete he'd always wanted to be. For James, there was Before Surgery and After Surgery.

As promised from his hospital bed at age fourteen, James had started donating blood at eighteen, the legal minimum age in Australia. He went to donor mobiles—large converted school buses first called into use in Australia in 1942—whenever they rolled into town, meeting different nurses and doctors with each visit. But when he got a promotion working in the accounting and clerical department at the railway and was relocated to Sydney, he found a home of sorts in the Red Cross blood bank at 1 York Street.

James admired the camaraderie there: Recipes were traded, gardening tips shared, friendships formed, and birthdays and anniversaries remembered. There were husbands and wives and fathers and sons who donated together. No one was paid a dime for their blood.

The Red Cross blood center building had a rich history, beginning its life as the manor home of Dr. Dunmore Lang, a famous Presbyterian minister in colonial days. It then became the storied Petty's Hotel for more than a century and served during World War II as housing for Royal Navy officers. The New South Wales division of the Red Cross bought the building in 1950, shuttered the hotel, and opened the center in 1952.

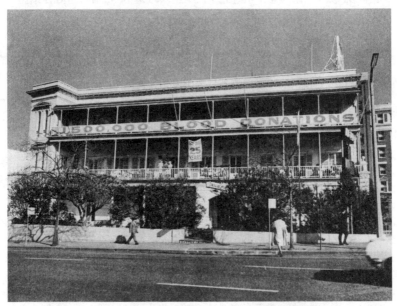

The Red Cross Blood Transfusion Service building
at 1 York Street on Church Hill in Sydney, Australia.

James was settling into his new life in Sydney. He'd taken exams for three possible careers straight out of high school: in banking, public service, and the railways. When he learned that working for the railroad was the only profession that wouldn't require him to work weekends, his choice was made. He wanted weekends free to play sports.

The Commonwealth Railways gave employees paid time off to donate blood. James's father, Reginald, also a regular blood donor, went to the donor mobile whenever he could. Australia never paid donors for blood; donating was just a way of life, like sheep shearing in the spring, the wheat harvest in the fall, or the constant whistle of trains.

The clerical job suited James. He took pride in never being particularly ambitious. He viewed work as a way to provide "three square meals a day and keep the wolf from the door." He liked playing cards and sports on the weekends, listening to country music, and watching trains pass by. The train station in Sydney was beautiful and bustling and had lines taking passengers anywhere they wanted to go. James was working his way up the job ladder, but happy and patient with every step. He recruited his colleagues in Sydney to donate blood with him.

In the blood bank's cramped donor room, the nurse hit James's vein on the first try.

"James," she said, "you have the loveliest veins."

"That's right—veins of steel," he said with pride.

James was also beaming about an important new development in his life. His lifelong friend Barbara Lindbeck had recently become his fiancée. The nurses loved to ask James, "How's the future Mrs. Harrison?"

James would never forget the day he realized Barb was more than a friend. She'd been away with her cousins in Sydney and was returning home days before the start of school. James, who was working as an apprentice bookkeeper at the railway in Junee at the time, had offered to pick her up. It was early morning, and James waited on the platform, watching the train from Sydney pull in and come to a stop. Passengers disembarked, but no Barbara. Suddenly, there in front of him stood Barb—now transformed into a beautiful young woman. *"She's not a bad sort at all, now is she?"* James thought. She wore a skirt, a fitted cardigan, and lipstick. When she kissed him on the cheek, he blushed as red as her sweater.

Growing up, Barb had been as fearless as any kid in town, riding her horse to school and joining in all of the boys' games. She always looked out for James in his early years when he was weak from illness.

Now they were both working in Sydney—Barb had taken a job teaching home economics in a high school—and regularly returned to Junee by train to see their families. She treasured James's oddball humor and kindness. He helped anyone in need, stepped in as the town Santa Claus when his dad had to work, and organized food drives for the local church. James prided himself on giving people "a fair shake of the sauce bottle," Australian slang for giving someone the benefit of the doubt. Every time James headed off to donate blood, Barb pulled him close and called him her "gorgeous man." She gave him a note that read: "Beauty Tip: Being Good Makes You Gorgeous."

James started out donating blood every eight weeks, then every six weeks, then every four. The process took about an hour from start to finish, from the time he checked in at the front desk, had his medical file updated and blood pressure taken, to when the blood draw was completed. Each draw took up to 8 percent of his blood volume— around 470 milliliters. His body would replace the volume drawn within a day or two. He donated because it was what he had promised from his hospital bed, and because of his belief that he was helping others.

In the small donor room, the nurse left James for a spell, and another donor walked in. James smiled at the familiar face and reached out his hand, "Hello, Mrs. Semmler."

Olive Semmler had a gentle smile, prematurely graying brown hair, and dark circles under her eyes. She sometimes arrived at the center with her daughter, Val, who worked at the nearby hospital and was a year younger than James. Chatty and cheerful one visit and taciturn and melancholy the next, she had shared with James occasional stories of her life: her gardens, fruit trees, and chickens. She was a farmer's wife—raising sheep and growing wheat—and lived hours away in the country town of Temora. She traveled over rough roads and in nasty weather to get to Sydney to donate blood.

Donating blood was simple for James, but he had learned it was much more complicated for many others, including Olive. He had heard the story of Olive's baby boy, who came into the world a few years after daughter Val was born in 1937. The boy's name was William Alexander, and he arrived looking beautiful and healthy, with his father's blue eyes and fair skin. But baby William never came home—he died four days after birth due to "blood complications." Olive was Rh negative and William was Rh positive. Even now, eighteen years later, Olive would not allow anyone to put a marker on William's grave. It was a finality she couldn't face. Olive told people, "I always wanted a blue-eyed boy."

James had come to realize that any discomfort he might go through in donating blood was nothing compared to the challenges faced by Olive and others he met at the blood bank. Many donors gave because of what they had lost. James donated because of what he'd been given.

James wanted to have a big family of his own one day and couldn't imagine the pain of losing a child. He also had questions about his friend Olive: *Why had her daughter, Val, been fine, when her son, William, wasn't?* He didn't know the answer, but her story of loss stayed with him. He would never have known by looking at Olive, always polite and impeccably dressed, that she had lived through such loss. She had suffered, and still managed to be kind. It was a lesson that James hoped he could carry for the rest of his life.

James and Olive were connected in a way that went beyond their dedication to donating, a way that was detectable only under a microscope. James's blood had unusually high levels of a certain antibody that could cause problems for transfusion recipients. Olive, it turned out, also had high levels of the antibody. Because of this, their blood was not suitable for human transfusions. It could only be used for research—not to save lives.

Over three years of donating, James had learned about basic blood typing. Though some of it went over his head, he understood there were eight main blood groups when including Rh positive and Rh negative, and that blood groups were identified by antibodies and antigens. Antibodies were Y-shaped molecules that neutralized antigens, like soldiers deployed to eliminate foreign invaders.

But as James finished his blood draw that day—he would get a glass of juice and a biscuit before going back to work—he wasn't worried in the least about his antigens or antibodies or about where his donated blood went. Sure, he would have liked to see his blood used for life-saving transfusions—to save lives the way he had been saved. But he believed in giving to give, without expecting anything in return. He didn't have money to donate. He wasn't a person of power or influence. But he had blood. All he had to do was sit back, roll up his sleeve, and extend his right arm.

CHAPTER FOUR
Life Is a Mystery

The mechanism of Rh disease—also called hemolytic disease of the newborn or *erythroblastosis fetalis*—had been understood since the late 1930s, when Vince Freda's mentor, Alexander Wiener discovered that the Rh factor was a type of protein, or antigen, on the surface of red blood cells. And researcher Philip Levine had unraveled the mechanism of Rh disease, finding that maternal Rh antibodies were responsible for harming Rh-positive babies who had inherited the Rh factor from the father. The findings were published in 1940, and there was a fierce and public rivalry between Wiener and Levine over who was more significant in the discovery and understanding of Rh disease, providing major drama at blood bank meetings for many years.

But nearly two decades after Wiener and Levine first published, there remained more questions than answers. One of the areas of research was looking into why the first Rh-positive baby born to an Rh-negative mother was spared when later pregnancies ended in loss. The thinking was that the first baby was born before antibodies appear, because a mother's primary immune response can take three months after delivery to develop. But in later pregnancies, there is a "secondary immune response," which is rapid. The question was how to prevent the occurrence of antibodies in Rh-negative mothers with Rh-positive babies.

Freda and Gorman had searched the records on 3x5 cards of hundreds of Rh patients. They wanted to study the natural history of Rh antibody levels in all the Rh mothers seen at Columbia and tested in the Presbyterian Hospital blood bank. Now, Gorman drew and erased and scribbled some more until his blackboard resembled a football playbook, with X's and O's and lines and arrows moving in different directions. In this case, though, offense and defense were mother and child.

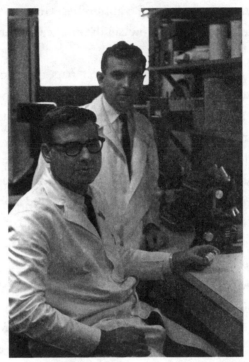

John Gorman (standing) with Dr. Vince Freda in the lab at Columbia.

Gorman's diagram was part of the latest brainstorming session between the young physician and Freda in Gorman's office at Columbia Presbyterian Hospital in Washington Heights. The diagram detailed how the immune system of a pregnant woman with Rh-negative blood perceives a threat from her unborn child who has Rh-positive blood. The mother deploys her antibodies through the placenta to defeat the antigens from the baby.

"Red cells are the sole target of the maternal Rh antibody," Gorman said, drawing more circles and arrows to show the damage to the fetus—the anemia, hypoxia, fetal edema, massive swelling of fetal liver and spleen, and inadequate fetal placental circulation, which could result in brain damage or death. The harm to the fetus depended on the intensity of the antibodies. Gorman asked, "Can one of the arrows be broken? How can the mother's immune response be stopped?"

Gorman and Freda read every research paper they could get their hands on, attended conferences, and met with immunologists and serologists, those assessing blood incompatibility for transfusions. But no one knew how to stop or limit an immunologic response in the mother. Could a mother be rendered unresponsive to the blood of her fetus? Several approaches were debated and tested. Babies were delivered early to mitigate the damage to the mother's red blood cells. This brought success and failure—failure when babies died of prematurity. Other approaches included giving mothers high doses of vitamin C, cortisone injections, and hormones. Nothing was working.

Freda had just opened an Rh Clinic at Columbia where all Rh-negative mother's pregnancies were managed to study the natural history of the disease. Rh-antibody concentrations were monitored closely, as was bilirubin in the amniotic fluid, to time early induction. Extra bilirubin was produced when a baby's red cells were being destroyed, and high levels of neonatal bilirubin were known to cause brain damage. Freda tracked the titer and bilirubin levels to extend a high-risk pregnancy for as long as possible.

Gorman wiped the board with the sleeve of his lab coat and scribbled on. Freda, always sleep deprived, always motivated, wondered whether it was possible to flood the mother's circulation with large amounts of antibodies to stop her from making her own antibodies. Other ideas included injecting the mother with large amounts of harmless antigen to try to distract her immune system from making the anti-Rh antibodies. This was a kind of "competition of antigens" approach, stimulating the body with other antigens in hopes of lowering the intensity of the mother's immune response.

Gorman scribbled "homeostasis," on the board, and thought through the body's ability to constantly regulate everything from blood sugar to calcium levels. "If you administer a thyroid extract injection, the body says, 'I won't make anymore,' because it knows it has enough thyroid hormones," Gorman noted. The body responds to excess by turning off the corresponding gland or organ.

Gorman and Freda had been in contact with research teams in England, Canada, and Australia who were working through similar ideas, experiments, and challenges to unravel the mystery of treating Rh disease and related immunological challenges. Gorman had become particularly interested in studies by another Australian doctor, Macfarlane Burnet, and British zoologist Peter Medawar, involving immunologic tolerance. Medawar's focus was on transplant rejections in animals and skin graft rejections by burn victims. He experimented first on rabbits by transplanting a patch of fur from one rabbit onto a different type of rabbit. The transplant rejection, he concluded, was an immune reaction. Medawar found that repetitive grafts from the same donor were rejected faster with each successive attempt. He began to work with mice in utero and found there was a "short immunologic null period," in utero and shortly after birth, when the immune system of a white mouse could be made to accept rather than reject skin transplants from a black mouse. The white mice were injected while still in utero with the bone marrow of the black mice. Remarkably, the white mice that had received the black mice's bone marrow accepted grafts or organs from the black mice throughout their lifetimes. The mice became immunologically tolerant to the foreign antigens.

"What we need to do is to make the mother tolerant to the Rh in the baby," Gorman said, aware of the considerable leap from studies on mice to studies on pregnant women.

Gorman and Freda would continue like this for hours, presenting, supporting, debunking. Gorman had become fixated on his own theory of immunological tolerance that he believed explained why the white mice didn't reject the foreign black mice skin. He believed that there were cells in one's immune system that were benign and did no harm. "Tolerance is an active immune response," Gorman deduced. "The lymphocytes responding during the null period were immunologically incompetent or tolerant cells that didn't harm you." But when Gorman first proposed that these benign cells had to exist to explain immunological tolerance, colleagues didn't buy it. His theories were soundly dismissed.

After a lively back and forth brainstorming with Freda, Gorman concluded their latest session. The young doctor spent most of his waking hours on the Rh mystery, but in recent months, he had started dealing with another kind of mystery—one that was also very difficult to solve.

The puzzle came in the form of a certain resident who worked in the adjacent blood bank. The resident had long blonde hair, lovely blue eyes, a midwestern twang, and a way with patients. Her name was Carol Rutgers, and she was a pathology resident working in the blood bank three days a week, earning $5 an hour drawing blood to be stored in glass bottles. She'd arrived at Columbia from the University of Chicago Medical School, where she was a top student, having aced her medical college admission exam, and was one of only six women in her class of seventy-two. She was a mix of confident and nurturing, and men of all ages swooned in her presence. She received marriage proposals like compliments. Carol, looking up from her work at the blood bank, saw John smiling bashfully from across the room.

Carol had landed in the blood center shortly after starting her four-year residency at Columbia. She had been told, "The director needs someone in there to help." So she began dividing her time between the blood bank and classes. She got along well with the director, John Scudder, a pioneer in blood banks who was a part of the mission begun by Charles Drew to get American plasma to British soldiers during the early years of World War II. Scudder had helped establish the blood bank at Presbyterian Hospital in 1939 as one of the first three to open in the United States. He had made Gorman his assistant director and championed Gorman's keen mind.

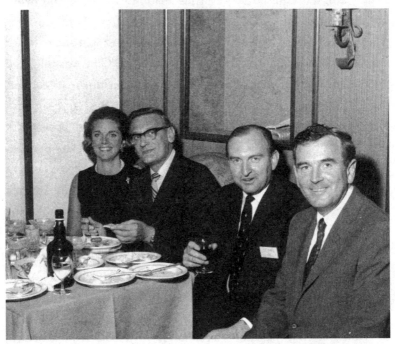

From far right: John Gorman with unknown colleague, chemist Bill Pollack, and Carol Freda, Vince Freda's wife.

Carol liked John from the day they met. She found him attractive, with his dark curly hair and gray-blue eyes. When they started dating, though, she wondered whether he'd ever been out with girls before. He acted nervous and flustered, and she could only understand about half of what he said. His Australian accent was adorable—but hard to decipher. She admired his loyalty to his family in Australia and was impressed that he came from a family of doctors. Two of his siblings were in medical school, and his other sister was studying law.

John and Carol took in Broadway shows and tried out new restaurants, often double dating with Vince and his wife—whose name was also Carol. They especially loved the remake of the musical *Show Boat*. Carol was amused by John's fascination with cars—and by his misadventures with cars. His first car, the light green Ford, was long gone. He had parked it on a street in Manhattan one night and returned after dinner to find it wouldn't start. "It's no good," he was told, and reluctantly abandoned it. When his next car broke down in Manhattan, he left it for a day or two. When he returned, the car was picked clean—a sad sight for a machine he loved. He then bought a beautiful two-door, two-tone 1954 Oldsmobile coup, green on the bottom, beige on top. The fate of this car was no better. It was totaled one night in a hit and run while parked on the street. At one point, Gorman bought a ten-year-old Studebaker for $50. It had a good run, outlasting the others.

It soon became apparent to colleagues at Columbia that John and Carol were an item. Dr. Scudder and his wife began inviting the young couple to their gorgeous weekend home on Shelter Island, where they would spend the day sailing. John shared with Carol stories of Scudder's unexpected ways, telling Carol how he dreaded driving with him, especially when they were leaving Scudder's home on 120th Street in Manhattan. Scudder loved to tear out of his garage, careen around the corner, and then blast up and onto Broadway—all in a continuous acceleration that left John terrified and clutching his seat.

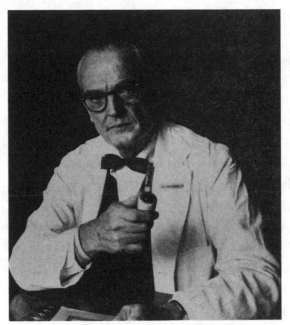

Blood pioneer and Columbia's blood bank director John Scudder, 1959.

Carol had already concluded that Columbia attracted eccentric and brilliant minds. She learned early on in their courtship not to take it personally when John drifted off mid-conversation. He was polite and kind, and she knew he was trying to listen. He would look her in the eyes when she was talking, but she knew his mind was elsewhere, back in the lab solving some complex problem. She told a girlfriend: "He's a total genius, there's no doubt about that."

But as the months dragged on—with no solution to Rh disease in sight—Gorman wasn't feeling like a total genius. The X's and O's on the chalkboard were beginning to feel more like scribbles than strategy, and he was becoming frustrated beyond words. In his youth, there had been the math challenges, the nonlinear differential equations, equations with co-prime integers and inverse functions, followed a few years later by his exploration into number theory.

These days, however, he was consumed with a vexing set of numbers that were the opposite of sublime. The numbers played over in his mind, wherever he was. By the late 1950s, more than two hundred thousand babies were dying each year from Rh disease, according to developed countries that collected and reported the data. Perhaps twice that many lived but suffered brain damage and other irreversible impairments. The United States alone was reporting forty thousand cases of Rh disease annually, with ten thousand babies lost every year to the affliction. It was an astonishing, horrifying amount of loss and suffering.

The Rh problem was even worse in Australia, as the disease was especially common among families of Irish, English, and Scottish descent who made up most of Australia's population. In Australia, Rh potentially affected one in six newborns. *One in six.* Gorman still lived with the memory of the baby whom he had watched die in the operating room in Melbourne. It was an awful thing to witness. At the same time, it was an image he had probably needed to see as a medical student. A helpless newborn subjected to hours of surgical interventions through the night, only to die on the table in the early morning hours.

The days passed and the search continued. Gorman sat at his desk and looked out across the shimmering Hudson River. Over to the right, construction of the second deck of the George Washington Bridge was underway. The buildings and the gray sky blended into a gradual fade. There were days when doubt crept into his mind over his decision to come to America. He had been so optimistic when he set sail for America—holding onto the streamer connected to his mother for as long as he could. Was it the naivete of youth that made him believe he could make a name for himself in the United States?

Gorman contemplated his fate. He had his beautiful girlfriend, Carol—mysterious as women might be—and he'd developed a nice group of friends here. But he had not come to America to improve his social life. In the competitive petri dish that was Columbia, he felt impatient watching others succeed. He was not accustomed to answers that remained elusive.

CHAPTER FIVE
The Hobby of Happiness

James admired the fiery sunset over the Great Smoky Mountains along the Tennessee–North Carolina border. Next he studied a pastoral farm with giant rolls of hay in Lancaster, Pennsylvania. Then he traveled to the Rio Grande in Texas, and quickly on to the snow-dusted peaks of Mount McKinley in Alaska. Finally, his gaze settled on the gorgeous layered bands of red rocks in the Grand Canyon in Arizona.

James was on a train traveling to Sydney. By his side was Barb, his plucky childhood friend who was now his wife. The newlyweds had been to Junee to visit their families. Now, to pass the time, James pulled a red binder from his bag and formally invited his wife to "travel the world" with him. They traveled this way—through America, Europe, the Far East, and beyond—by his stamp collection, which he'd started when he was five years old and arranged by continent, country, region, city, year, and subject. These small pieces of affixable paper were his portals to the wider world.

James and Barb were saving to buy a house, so stamps were all the escape they could afford. James's collection encompassed everything: geography, movies, music, science, technology, space, sports, celebrities, events, religion, and more. It also presented its share of inventory challenges. "It's annoying when these countries in Africa keep changing their names and you don't know where to put them," James said. He also couldn't understand the lack of uniformity in the size of Eastern European stamps.

The stamps were about past and present. They were about the rhythms of a day, whether ephemeral, rich, or momentous. The collection was biographical, starting with stamps reflecting James's childhood interests in kangaroos, koala bears, and King George V. Barb was drawn in, too, but her attraction was the romanticism of the letters that these stamps enabled. She imagined words of solace and love, and simple stories of everyday lives, dropped into mailboxes and opened with joy, concern, or curiosity. James spent hours putting together new albums, carefully placing stamps onto black pages with special tongs, and then slowly flipping through the pages to admire his work. At a glance, the pages were a mosaic. Up close, there was a narrative.

As the train sped along toward Sydney, the newlyweds continued their travel across America, taking in the Statue of Liberty, the White House, the Lincoln Memorial, the Washington Monument, and the Golden Gate Bridge.

James and Barb enjoyed their visits to Junee, though for James, everything was so much smaller than he remembered it as a child. The family home. His school. The distance from his driveway to the train tracks, where he would race. His family home at 32 Pitt Street was unchanged: white clapboard siding, paned windows, red roof, front porch with old chairs, and a small yard enclosed by wire fencing. The family didn't have a lot of money, but James and his sister never wanted for anything. His father, Reginald, had recently been put in charge of the machine shop that made sure the wheels of the locomotives ran safely and efficiently.

Barb looked at her watch and reminded James to drink his water. "Three glasses of water two hours before you donate, right?" she said. They were over halfway through the six-hour ride back to Sydney.

James tried not to miss a visit to the Red Cross center at 1 York Street. Today, Barb would head home and James would visit the center on his own. Barb had the day off from teaching, and James would play catchup at work later that night.

With hours remaining on the train ride, James returned to his stamp collection. Most collectors loved rarities, firsts, and errors and only wanted the "mint" stamps, those straight from the post office and never used. But James thought the stamps with little tears, folds, and imperfections added rich details to the story, like years and wrinkles would add character to the people he loved. He was sure that Barb at forty would be even more beautiful than Barb at twenty.

Barb looked for stamps with animals and anything to do with horses. Even though she and James now lived in Sydney, she would always be a country girl at heart. James had spent many weekends helping his father-in-law by chasing sheep and lumping bags of wheat on his shoulders. Barb's parents had looked after James's family during World War II, bringing them precious homemade butter and other provisions from their farm. When James's dad had first arrived in Junee to work for the railway, Barb's father was the welcoming party, introducing Reginald around and making him feel like a part of the community. His parents and Barb's still played cards together every weekend.

The rest of the trip to Sydney passed quickly. James and Barb chuckled at the names of the towns they sped through: Galong, Binalong, Oolong, Tallong. When they hit Erskineville, they knew they were close. They soon arrived at the gorgeous Sydney Town Hall station, built with brick and local sandstone and with thick windows that filtered light in fat golden beams. Barb and James paused to listen to an energetic ukulele band on a nearby platform. When they parted ways, Barb kissed him and said, "You're a gorgeous man, James Harrison."

It's a simple life, but a good life, James thought to himself as he boarded a bus to 1 York Street, fast becoming his home away from home.

CHAPTER SIX
The Ferrets Sneezed!

After eating lunch in the downstairs cafeteria at Columbia, John Gorman headed back to the lab. He had work to do in the blood bank, not to mention new pet projects: tinkering with various inventions in different stages of development. Because the Rh conundrum still seemed as unsolvable as ever, Gorman was doing a lot of tinkering, not only as a side pursuit, but also as a sort of therapy for his slow-going Rh research. If he wasn't going to make a name for himself as a doctor, he was determined to make a name—and maybe even a fortune—as an inventor.

One of Gorman's first product overhauls at Columbia Presbyterian involved the prothrombin time test used to measure how quickly a patient's blood clots. Gorman took one look at the crazy Rube Goldberg–like contraption and knew he could do better. The prothrombin test was widely used in clinical labs and hospitals for everything from diagnosing liver problems and assessing the body's ability to clot during surgery, to monitoring the effectiveness of blood-thinning medications.

The machine at Columbia, though, was a jerry-rigged hobbyist fish tank with a standard aquarium heater to keep the water at 95 degrees Fahrenheit (37°C). A metal rack immersed test tubes to keep blood samples warm. There was a stopwatch involved, and various wires and threads to test the sticky plasma. Gorman thought, *This is how we are saving lives?* It got worse: To run the test, the technician had to use a mouth pipette to suck plasma up and then back into the tube. Technicians—including Gorman—had accidents when small amounts of the blood were sucked into their mouth.

So, Gorman began building his own prothrombin machine by rigging vacuum tubes, a small amplifier, and a photocell. Many of the pieces he cobbled together had been left over from the Manhattan Project, the work during World War II at Columbia and elsewhere to develop the first nuclear weapons.

A few weeks after Gorman had version one of his new makeshift machine, one of the medical device salesmen who regularly came by spotted the contraption. On the next visit, the salesman told Gorman that his medical company would give him $2,500 to buy better equipment to build a better machine. The second iteration was built, and soon Gorman and a partner had formed a medical-laboratory automation company. The hunt for the next invention always gave Gorman a rush, yet it was difficult to ease his frustration over his lack of progress on Rh disease.

It was not lost on the competitive Gorman that Melbourne—where he'd gone to medical school—had since his departure become a leading center of immunologic research. The credit for the notoriety Down Under had gone to renowned virologist Macfarlane Burnet. Burnet, though shy like Gorman, was a master of garnering attention, and had impressed Australians by turning down the offer of a prestigious departmental chair at Harvard to stay in Melbourne. Most important, Burnet had captivated the scientific community with his clonal selection theory of immunity, postulating that every cell in a body descends from a single cell. His microevolutionary explanation of the nature of antibody production heralded a new era in immunology. Burnet explained tolerance by asserting that the immune cells that could respond to self were *deleted* in the thymus during the null period, thus preventing autoimmunity. This meant that there were no cells left that could make autoimmune antibodies.

Gorman's own theory on immunological tolerance—his ideas around the work of benign cells—had basically asserted the opposite.

He believed there were cells that started as clones, as Burnet theorized, but were not antibody producing. Instead, these small lymphocytes—a form of white blood cell—didn't make antibodies. "They are 'tolerant' cells," Gorman noted. "Tolerance is an active response." Just as Burnet's theory was unanimously applauded, Gorman's conclusions were unanimously dismissed. Of course, Burnet was *Sir Macfarlane Burnet*. He had been knighted for his studies on the capacity of organisms to distinguish between "self" and "not self" and for the development of techniques to grow the influenza virus in a chick embryo. His theories were widely published, and his comings and goings made news. While visiting a lab in London that was the first to transmit the human influenza virus to animals, he was in the hallway when he heard a scientist yelling excitedly: "The ferrets sneezed, the ferrets sneezed!" Burnet would tell the story later and urge young scientists to hope for their own "the ferrets sneezed" moment to happen even once in their career. Burnet was now a contender for the Nobel Prize for his work on immunological tolerance, developed with Peter Medawar, who conducted the experiments involving skin grafts from black mice to white mice.

Gorman looked at his watch and grabbed his lab uniform. It was time to help second-year medical students in their tissue pathology class. His job was to walk from student to student, answering questions and offering observations on the tissue specimens representing different kinds of pathology, from carcinoma of the pancreas to tuberculosis in the lung. The specimens had come from autopsies and surgeries and represented common diseases.

As the class wound down and students dispersed, Gorman spotted one of the regular book salesmen enter the lab, chat up the students, and head his way. The salesman was from W. B. Saunders Company, and he stopped by regularly, hoping that professors would select his books for class adoption or that students would buy copies. The salesman told

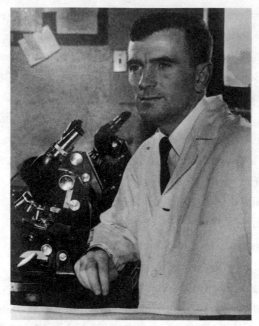

John Gorman as a resident in the blood bank at Columbia.

Gorman that he wanted to give him a complimentary, hot-off-the-press copy of the second edition of *General Pathology*, a textbook edited by none other than Sir Howard Florey, a famous Australian scientist who shared the Nobel Prize for his involvement in the development of penicillin. The book was based on lectures delivered in the school of pathology at Oxford.

"This is great," Gorman said, enthusiastically flipping through the heavy red textbook—nearly one thousand pages—which covered everything from the history and scope of pathology and the reactions of blood to injuries to the biological factors in the production of antibodies. Gorman and the salesman soon parted ways, and Gorman headed back to his office.

Sitting at his desk, he leafed through the new pathology book and began to scan the chapters, reading short passages on hemorrhage and shock and the effects of injury on metabolism. He flipped back to the table of contents and then forward to Chapter 34, page 697. The chapter was titled, "Biological Factors in the Production of Antibodies."

Gorman began reading: "The antibody response of an animal receiving an antigenic stimulus for the first time differed considerably from that of an animal which had previously encountered the antigen."

He continued reading until one sentence gave him pause:

"The presence of circulating antibody, whether produced actively or received passively, depresses and may completely inhibit the immune response to the relevant antigen, although not to other antigens."

Gorman moved his index finger under the text, reading it again—and then again. The author was focused on the immune response in test animals. Gorman was thinking of Rh disease in humans.

This is beautiful in its simplicity, Gorman thought, pushing back from his desk and beginning to pace. He rifled through piles of papers before turning to the files in his cabinets. He found what he was looking for: a research paper titled, "Active Immunity Produced by So-Called Balanced or Neutral Mixtures of Diphtheria Toxin and Antitoxin." The paper was written in 1909 by Theobald Smith, an American microbiologist and pathologist who had been called a "microbe hunter."

Smith's applied research studies involved toxins (antigens) and antitoxins (antibodies) as a vaccine for diphtheria. Smith varied the ratio of the antigens to the responding antibody in tests on guinea pigs. In the 1909 paper—written less than a decade after the three major human blood groups were discovered by Landsteiner—Smith found that he could *protect* guinea pigs from getting diphtheria by giving them high doses of the antibody produced in response to the presence of the bacteria. The finding suggested that instead of waiting for the guinea pig to develop diphtheria, one could inject the animal with antibodies from another animal responding to the same toxin. These were "passive antibodies," because the animal didn't actively make the antibodies itself. Gorman thought about this: Would the immune system filled with passive antibodies feel adequately protected and not launch its own defense?

Gorman continued reading: "From the practical standpoint it offers a promising field for investigations in the active immunization of the human subject."

Smith went on: "The foregoing and earlier data taken together demonstrate that an active immunity lasting several years can be produced in guinea pigs, by the injection of toxin-antitoxin mixtures which have no recognizable harmful effect. They also show [that an] excess of antitoxin reduces the possibility of producing an active immunity and may extinguish it altogether."

Gorman went back over this sentence: *An excess of antibody reduces the possibility of producing an active immunity and may extinguish it altogether.*

Gorman was captivated by the four last words: *may extinguish it altogether.*

The field of immunology from its inception had been focused on how to make a *better* immune response. Gorman and Freda had been banging their heads against a wall trying to figure out how to *stop* an immune response. Gorman had gone over and over the blood bank records of hundreds of women who had suffered losses because of Rh disease. He felt like a detective returning to a crime scene, certain he had missed one critical piece of evidence.

Standing in his office—which now looked like a small tornado had rolled through—Gorman thought: *The solution is the problem.* Give the mother passive antibodies so she doesn't produce her own antibodies. Fool her immune system into thinking that it already has responded to the Rh antigen. It was not lost on Gorman that the same substance that was killing the babies could be the medicine that prevented the disease.

Gorman grabbed the *General Pathology* textbook and dashed out of his office. He needed to find Vince Freda.

Darting through the hospital corridors, Gorman spotted Freda talking with a patient. Freda could see that his friend was worked up over something.

"I've got it!" Gorman exclaimed, barely waiting for Freda to finish with the patient. Gorman opened *General Pathology* and flipped through the pages. He found his highlighted sentences and began to read aloud:

The presence of circulating antibody, whether produced actively or received passively, depresses and may completely inhibit the immune response to the relevant antigen, although not to other antigens.

Then he produced Smith's paper and read a short passage: *An excess of antibody reduces the possibility of producing an active immunity and may extinguish it altogether.*

Freda nodded. He was working through the mechanisms of the idea.

"This is it," Gorman said. "This is how we stop Rh disease."

"This is an *un*-vaccine or the *anti*-vaccine," Gorman said, referring to how vaccines work by training an immune response to recognize and combat viruses or bacteria. The treatment for Rh would be to *prevent immunity*, to inhibit the active antibody response that would harm the baby.

Gorman studied Freda's face. Freda got it. But Gorman also knew that Freda was desperate to find something, anything, that would work for Rh. Freda had been dealing with the death of Rh babies and the grief of families for too long.

Gorman continued, "We inject the Rh-negative mother with the same antibody that she would naturally produce when hit with the Rh-positive blood of her fetus."

Freda said, "So the very thing known to kill babies is their salvation."

The difference was in intensity, Gorman noted. The injected antibody would be just strong enough to prevent the mother from making
an immune response but not strong enough to harm the baby. Or so
he theorized.

The men looked at each other and smiled. This was their moment.
The ferrets were sneezing.

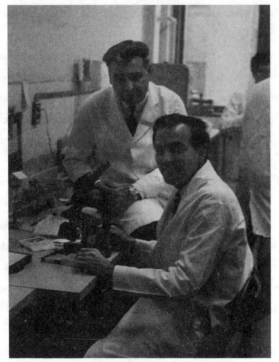

John Gorman (seated) with Vince Freda, working on
different ideas for how to combat Rh disease.

But as Gorman and Freda excitedly shared the idea around the hospital
and blood bank, they elicited a series of patronizing looks. Everyone
had the same response: "Oh, sure, you're going to give the pathological
antibodies that are killing the baby to the mother." Another popular
refrain was: "It's another of John's crazy ideas."

Even John's girlfriend, Carol, could understand the prevailing skepticism among his colleagues. "To the man on the street," she told him, "it does seem insane."

The medical establishment soon delivered the same verdict. The National Institutes of Health called the passive-antibody-as-treatment idea "a nonsense," and major funding bodies refused to support it. Everywhere Gorman and Freda turned, they ran into what Gorman called "a lot of nonbelievers."

Gorman was frustrated but understood the skepticism. People tended to shy away from the disruptive, even when it was good. He mused that it was probably traceable to Darwin's ideas around survival and a sense that it was better to go with something safe than take a risk on something new. Besides, most of those who dismissed the idea hadn't read the Florey textbook, and they hadn't read the original papers on the development of vaccines for diphtheria, tetanus, and polio. Scientists worked in silos, and information was not easily or readily shared. Besides, as he lamented with Freda one day, "You can tell people things, but they need to see the data and digest the data."

Undeterred, Gorman and Freda continued to apply for grants and talk up anyone who would listen. Gorman was awed by Freda's tenacity. As soon as one more grant application was denied, Freda was drafting another. One day, months into their crusade, they were invited to a talk being given by a well-regarded protein chemist named William Pollack of Ortho Pharmaceutical Co. Pollack, who Gorman thought was the spitting image of Michael Caine, British accent and all, came to Columbia to talk about the Coombs test, which checked blood for antibodies that attack red blood cells. Gorman and Freda tag-teamed Pollack after the talk to share their ideas on Rh. They had recently been turned down for support by none other than Philip Levine, who had discovered the mechanisms of Rh disease. Levine, who had started the center for blood group research at Ortho, didn't think Gorman and Freda's passive-antibody-as-solution approach would work. But William Pollack—miraculously—was receptive. The three men spent the rest of the afternoon holed up in Freda's lab.

Pollack, the son of a carpenter who had served in the Royal Navy during World War II and had bachelor's and master's degrees in chemistry, had earned a doctorate in zoology while researching Rh disease. In 1956, at the time he joined Ortho as director of research, Ortho Pharmaceutical was a subsidiary of Johnson & Johnson and best known for developing contraceptives, spermicidal jellies, and intrauterine devices. Pollack told Freda and Gorman that he began working on the fractionation of plasma into different protein components, another breakthrough developed during World War II. The technology was used by Edwin Cohn, a professor at Harvard Medical School, to separate human blood plasma into different components to treat wounded soldiers, including burn victims at Pearl Harbor. Pollack told Gorman and Freda that he could use fractionation to purify gamma globulin and isolate antibodies.

After all the jokes, the no's, the rejections, the general disbelief, here was not only a believer—but a possible enabler. Gorman could barely contain himself.

Gorman asked his next question tentatively: "Any chance you have Rh antibodies?"

Pollack responded: "I have a freezer full of the stuff."

CHAPTER SEVEN
The Downside of a Miracle

"Hello, Nurse Lizzie!" James said to the newest addition on the staff, Lizzie Thynne, who beamed when she saw James enter the Sydney blood bank. No matter the time of day, Lizzie always seemed to be at the front counter to check donors in. She'd retrieve charts, ask a series of questions, and then take donors to the back room to get them situated either in the chair that fully reclined or the one that required their legs to be extended out the window.

Lizzie had blue eyes, pale skin, and light brown hair pulled into a ponytail. She was one of the most guileless people James had ever met. She said anything that came to mind, and peppered people with questions. Lizzie had been a nurse in Brisbane before coming to Sydney. A friend told her, "Why don't you go to Sydney to work in the blood bank? I hear they need people and are doing interesting work." So she did.

"Let me get you checked in," Lizzie told James at the counter. She somehow managed to remember everything about James and the other donors. She knew he loved country music, that he and his new wife, Barb, were thinking of getting a dog, that he had a stamp collection, and that Barb worked long hours as a high school teacher.

When she had first met James, Lizzie had asked, "What brings you in here so regularly?"

"It's a habit, I suppose," James said. "And it feels like a family. Everyone knows you, everybody is friendly, and it doesn't hurt." He was also proud that Australia had one of the strongest traditions in volunteer blood donation, donating the second-largest quantity of blood in the world after the Swiss.

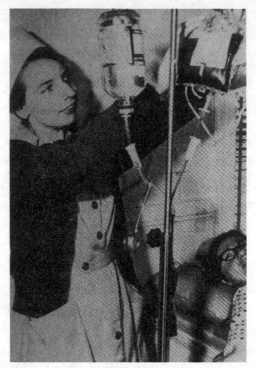

Nurse Lizzie Thynne works with a patient at the Red Cross center in Sydney, Australia.

James had taken to calling Lizzie a "sticky beak," an Australian term of endearment for someone who is chatty and asks a lot of questions. The term suited her in different ways, too. She had become known as the "bird lady," because of the birds she kept at home.

She told James, "When I iron, one of my chickens likes to stand there right on the ironing board and watch. I do quite a bit of talking to the chickens."

"I can only imagine," James said.

Like Olive Semmler and others James befriended at the blood bank, there was an emotional story buried under Lizzie's placid manner. Lizzie's mother had died giving birth to her. "I didn't have a mother, so I thought it would be nice to help other people in their sadness and times of distress," Lizzie told James one day. She had loved nursing from her first days on the job. She started out working in a maternity ward, caring for mothers and premature babies, including several babies with mysterious ailments that she now understood to be symptoms of Rh disease. She then worked in a home for developmentally disabled children while working the night shift at a nursing home.

During one of Lizzie's talks with James, when it was just the two of them in the donor room, he had asked her how someone got over the loss of a mother—at birth.

"Well, yes, everyone went to pieces," Lizzie said in her soft and lilting tone. "Daddy was a wreck. He couldn't think straight. He would go for a walk and get lost in the street. At first, no one knew what to do with me. I was going to be adopted out."

Lizzie continued, "My godmother took me in for six weeks, and the decision was made not to adopt me out. I was raised by my grand-mother. I never wanted to get married because I never wanted anyone to go through what my father went through."

Despite her circumstances, Lizzie always remained cheerful. "I was never a good student. My sister was the bright one. My dad would say, 'If you had the brains your sister had, you would go to university, too.' He was very proud of her. My grandmother sometimes told me that I should have died rather than my mother. I knew it was a loss for everyone. No one thought about my loss; I never had a mum. But I found my niche in nursing. I've been wonderfully happy. Blood, as they say, is thicker than water. My life is looking after all of you."

Monitoring the blood draw, Lizzie smiled at James and said, "Blood. You can't live without it, and you can't make it in a test tube. As soon as I arrived here, I knew I didn't need to go anywhere else."

Lizzie changed the subject, asking James, "Do you want one of my baby birds?" Lizzie had an aviary at home, and let her birds fly around her apartment. She offered chicks to regular donors.

"No, thank you!" James said with a laugh.

As James was finishing up, in walked Olive Semmler with her daughter, Val. Olive looked particularly melancholy today, so James tried to get her to smile by joking with Nurse Lizzie about her chicks and chickens. But Olive was in her own world, so James let her be.

As he stopped for his usual biscuit and tea on the way out, he saw Val and asked, "Is your mum okay?"

"She's alright," Val said. "It's an anniversary of one of the losses."

"Of the baby boy? William?"

"Oh, no, that was just the start," Val said. "William was the first loss. She and my father lost six more babies after William, all in a span of eleven years." Her parents had thought all the babies were fine, until they were delivered. Some arrived stillborn. Others, like William, succumbed after a few days of struggle.

"There was always the baby that never came home," Val said.

"*Seven* babies lost?" James asked. "Was it all the same blood problem you told me about?"

"Well, they didn't know about it at the time—my mum and dad always went to our little country hospital," Val said. "They should have come to Sydney. But now we are sure it was this problem with Rh, with blood type. My dad is Rh positive and my mum is Rh negative."

Val handed James a copy of a Red Cross pamphlet she was reading called *The Blood Donor*. The cover story was titled "Rh Factor is Not a Mystery." James read a few lines: "Most people have heard of Rh babies. These babies are born with anemia, and are sometimes yellow, or become yellow after birth. This is known as Hemolytic Disease of the Newborn."

Val said, "Apparently this disease—or curse—goes back to the beginning of time. The ancient Greeks described these symptoms of swollen babies, these yellow babies, babies brain damaged and babies that die after birth. But no one put a name to it until pretty recently."

"Is there a cure?" James asked.

"No, not yet—maybe one day," Val said.

For once, James was speechless. He had no idea that Olive had suffered so many losses. *Seven babies.* It was unthinkable. It made him even sadder for his friend and more appreciative of his own blessings. The gift of blood had supercharged his once weak body. Instead of fighting colds and catching every seasonal bug that came around, he was robust as ever, tossing hay, chasing sheep, and playing sports any chance he could get. On top of that, he was now happily married to the woman of his dreams. But for all his own good fortune, James could only watch as his friends at the blood bank suffered quietly.

Donating blood had begun to feel like his contribution to the world, his way of showing gratitude for how his life had been transformed. But he had learned that being supercharged with antibodies meant that his blood was destined for the research labs, not for people like Olive who needed it. He had convinced himself that simply giving blood was enough, but now he thought: *What good am I if I can't do good for others?*

CHAPTER EIGHT
Welcome to Sing Sing

John Gorman and Vince Freda could see their breath in the cold winter air as they waited to be buzzed into the heavily guarded confines of one of the nation's most notorious prisons, Sing Sing, situated on fifty-five acres overlooking the Hudson River in Ossining, New York. Guards with Thompson submachine guns manned the watchtowers, and the shouts of inmates and orders of guards echoed through the halls.

Gorman and Freda exchanged glances as they were buzzed in through the second set of gates, the heavy steel doors clanging shut behind them. The two doctors were now officially in the Big House, home to their first Rh trials with fractionated antibodies supplied by Bill Pollack at Ortho. The doctors were escorted into the office of Warden Wilfred Denno, a straight talker who liked to say he ran "the tightest ship on the Hudson." In the distance, behind the double bars on the semi-circular window in the warden's office, was the "Death House." This was headquarters of the "cee cees"—the condemned cells—and to the electric chair known as "Old Sparky," the dreaded site of more than six hundred executions.

Gorman and Freda were at Sing Sing on their own mission of life and death. They had recruited the lawless—including men who had taken lives—to do something that they hoped would save lives. Before the researchers could test Gorman's passive-antibody-as-immune-suppressor theory on pregnant women, the serum from Ortho would need to be tested on men. Prisoners were their proxy.

Until now, Gorman's only experience behind bars had been the few hours he had spent in the New York slammer after one of the nurses in the back seat of his car decided to pop her legs out the window just as police were driving by. He had seen movies said to be inspired by Sing Sing: *The Big House*, starring Robert Montgomery, and *Up the River*, starring Spencer Tracy and Humphrey Bogart. But nothing prepared him for this. The noise was the first jarring surprise. When Gorman and Freda walked in, inmates yelled out grievances. Clanging on the cell bars was another constant, along with the persistent buzzing of metal doors.

Warden Denno, who was strongly built, square-jawed, and unsmiling, said, "I was a young prison clerk at Auburn near Syracuse when we got caught up in a riot." Gorman's eyes widened. "I saw my coworker killed alongside of me, a deputy warden. That's a moment that stuck in my mind." Denno was now de facto dictator of the institution with about 1,800 prisoners and 500 employees. In 1951, a year after taking the job at Sing Sing, he had presided over four executions in one night.

The only advice Denno gave Gorman and Freda was: "Always be aware of your surroundings."

Gorman and Freda shook hands with the warden and headed out on a tour before being escorted to the prison hospital. The doctors were led through the halls of various buildings, mindful to stay to the right of the yellow lines for two-way walking. The warden thought they'd be interested in seeing the prison's Death House, and its electric chair. They were shown where last meals were prepared in the small kitchen next to the death chamber. Outside was a four-wall handball court. If a condemned man wanted to play, he had to compete against a guard.

"This is where America's first serial killer was put to death," the guard told Gorman and Freda. "Albert Fish was a child rapist and cannibal. He was executed here in 1936."

The guard added, "We had Ruth Snyder here. She was the first woman executed at Sing Sing. She murdered her husband with the help of her lover. The last person to sit in Old Sparky was Eddie Lee Mays, a robber and murderer." The guard said that the warden was sorting out the recent repeal of the death penalty by the state legislature for most capital crimes. Executions had been put on hold.

They were relieved when they were finally taken to the sick bay, where they were met by Dr. Harold Kipp, the prison's senior physician. Kipp, who had received his medical training at Columbia, had been instrumental in getting the skeptical Denno to approve the Rh study.

As they began to set up their equipment, Gorman looked over at his friend and colleague. Freda had been unrelenting in getting them here. He had spent a year lobbying the state attorney general and governor's office in Albany, writing grant applications, convincing the impassive Denno of the safety and merits of the study, and then drafting lengthy inmate consent forms. The NIH turned Freda down twice for funding, calling their reasoning "naïve." Bill Pollack of Ortho had also experienced his share of travails, testing various concentrations of the serum to be used in the trial before landing on one that he hoped was right. The truth was, though, no one knew optimal levels; they would have to learn as they went. After the NIH had turned down all financial requests, Gorman had managed to secure a $77,000 research grant from the Health Research Council, a new source of New York municipal funding. Gorman had been talking up the Rh idea with Donald McKay, Columbia's chair of pathology. When the council approached McKay to say they had funding for important new research, McKay steered them to Gorman and Freda.

When the trial was finally approved, it was Freda who had come to Sing Sing by himself to recruit inmates. Gorman knew that his idea was nothing without Freda's dogged determination. Flyers were circulated to prisoners, and Warden Denno made it clear that there were "no promises made, and no special favors offered" for this "entirely voluntary" program. Denno had been convinced by Gorman and Freda, and by his own prison doctor, that the tests were safe, and would be entirely different from some of the medical experiments involving inmates at other prisons that had taken healthy men and made them sick. "Not under my watch," Denno had said.

In a room filled with hundreds of inmates, Freda had delivered a speech that moved hardened criminals to tears. He told them of the struggles of Rh babies, of babies who arrived stillborn, and of the heartbreak of mothers and fathers. "We believe we are on the cusp of a breakthrough," Freda had said, adding emphatically, "You all can make a difference. You can save lives." He reassured the men that they could expect no side effects and no health problems. He made them laugh when he said, "The only danger would be if you plan to get pregnant." The biggest risk with any blood trial, he said, was hepatitis. But the fractionization at Ortho would mitigate the risk by taking whole blood and separating it into different parts.

One by one after Freda's talk, more than one hundred inmates came forward to have their blood tested to be a part of the trial. Overwhelmed by the response, Freda told the men he could only take donors with Rh-negative blood. Many of the inmates stopped to share stories of their own families, wives, and kids. A few wanted to know more about symptoms in a baby with Rh disease, saying they had lost babies of their own, but didn't know why. Inmate after inmate told Freda, "Whatever you need." As it turned out, thirty-six of the hundred-plus inmates were Rh negative and could be enrolled in the trial. The next step was to choose nine of the thirty-six for phase one of the trial.

Now that both Gorman and Freda had arrived in Sing Sing, the subjects of the study were gathering in the sick bay. The men, ranging in age from twenty-two to sixty-one, quietly lined up, were signed in, and instructed to take seats. Gorman separated the men into two groups, with four "treated" and five "controls." The treated were injected with 5 milliliters (1 teaspoon) of the Ortho passive antibody serum. The control group didn't get the serum. All nine men were then injected with 2 milliliters each of Rh-positive blood. Gorman opened his ledger and began to record notes in columns, showing dosage and injection dates. He wrote the inmate's first initial and last name: A. Curran; J. Fox; L. Hayden; A. Lobello; W. Asher; A. Burton; S. Young; F. Leonardis, and D. Maldonado.

As Gorman made more entries in the ledger, an inmate approached and asked him if he needed help with record keeping.

Gorman wasn't sure what to say.

"I'd be happy to do that for you," the inmate continued.

Gorman asked, "And what do you do? I mean, before you got here?"

"I'm an accountant," the man said. Gorman had to chuckle.

"Let's give it a try," Gorman said, noting that he would need exact dosage amounts, and blood draw times and amounts.

On the way out that day, carrying a cooler with serum and blood, Gorman said to Freda, "Sure different from what I expected. I mean, these guys are polite. That one fellow is an accountant!"

Freda knew that Gorman, consumed with ideas, theories, and inventions, was something of an innocent in the world. He warned him, "Don't get too comfortable. They're in here for a reason."

Gorman nodded and said, "One inmate kept telling me, 'Don't do the crime if you can't do the time.'"

Freda smiled. He had met his share of good guys and hustlers, heroes and fakes. He grew up in New Jersey, where his father worked for a company that designed uniforms, and had graduated from Columbia University in three years to spare his parents a fourth year of tuition. He'd worked his way through New York University medical school, and was drafted into the Air Force, serving out the tail end of the Korean War in Japan as a doctor to U.S. pilots. He went in as a lieutenant and came out as a captain, commended for his contribution to the understanding of optimal oxygen levels for pilots. Freda never wanted to be anything but a doctor.

On the forty-minute drive from Sing Sing back to Manhattan, Gorman and Freda started a new routine of stopping for lunch at a restaurant with a view of the water. Vince and his wife, Carol, had recently had their first child, a girl named Pamela, and Freda was besotted. Freda and Gorman ordered martinis, took in the view, and gave thanks that they were free men and could come and go from the Big House.

Inevitably their talk would return to the subject of blood and Rh. While both men believed that passive antibodies would work to stop Rh disease, they couldn't agree on how it would work at a molecular level. Would the fetal red cells be *cleared* by the passive antibodies? Would *cloaking* the antigens stop the immune system from producing its own antibodies? Would the body's homeostasis—or equilibrium system—kick in, telling the immune system it already had enough of something? Was it possible to get immune suppression without clearing the cells? Gorman kept returning to that one sentence from *General Pathology*: "An excess of antibody reduces the possibility of producing an active immunity and may extinguish it altogether."

As the men sipped their martinis, they savored their hard-fought victory of just getting their Sing Sing trials up and running. The process had been almost as frustrating as their path to the contrarian and ridiculed idea of giving passive Rh antibodies as a protection against Rh-positive antigens. For months on end, they had been on this roller coaster of sleepless nights, bright ideas, missed clues, breakthroughs, false alarms, depression, calculation, cooperation, and ridicule. They had come to realize that this was the status quo of modern medical inquiries, a continuum of tedium, euphoria, missteps, and incremental advances.

In setting up the trial, Freda and Gorman had laid out three steps: show that carefully calibrated doses of passive antibody prevent an active immune response—and apply it to Rh-negative male volunteers to show they could be protected from Rh immunization by passive antibody; develop a practical and safe method of providing passive Rh antibody in a larger group of Rh-negative males; and eventually start a trial of passive antibody in Rh-negative mothers at risk in the Rh clinic at Columbia.

Gorman and Freda were increasingly aware of other Rh trials and experiments racing ahead with equal fervor. There was a group in Liverpool, England, led by Cyril Clarke and Ronnie Finn, that was testing antibodies out on a dozen Rh-negative male policemen. Impressive work was being done by Canadian doctors Alvin Zipursky and Bruce Chown. An ob/byn named Eugene Hamilton in St. Louis, Missouri, was reportedly making his own anti-Rh formula, taking the blood of Rh-negative women who had delivered stillborn or moribund babies and had high concentrations of anti-Rh antibodies and injecting the blood into pregnant women at risk. There were also German workers testing their ideas out on Rh-negative male volunteers.

"This is the Rh college," Gorman said of the many doctors and researchers across the globe who were working on various ideas to eradicate the disease. All had the same idea of using passive antibodies to stop an active immune response. Beginning with the work of Philip Levine, it had been clear that if the mother did not get sensitized, the babies would be fine. As Gorman said, "Everyone understood if you could prevent the mother from getting sensitized—getting immunized and developing the antibodies herself—the disease could be halted."

The researchers shared a belief that passive antibodies would do the trick, and now just needed to prove it. There was debate over whether the Brits' crew or Gorman and Freda came up with the idea first. One story even had it that Cyril Clarke's wife awoke in the middle of the night and said, "Give them antibodies!" Gorman believed that lab work by Ronnie Finn had been the most instrumental in advancing their ideas. It had been Finn who had used the Kleihauer–Betke test, or acid elution test, invented by Enno Kleihauer and Klaus Betke in Germany in 1957, to determine the number of fetal cells present in the mother's blood. Finn discovered that the more fetal cells circulating in the mother's blood, the more risk to the baby. Finn spent months on the arduous test, which required visual counts of cells. Day after day, he measured the precise amounts of blood, treated it with reagents, and smeared it onto a gridded slide. He then had to count the number of cells in each grid box, looking at red cells, white cells, maternal cells, and fetal cells—which looked different than the maternal cells.

"The solitary inventor is a myth," Gorman said to Freda over lunch, taking in the view of the water. "Invention happens simultaneously and incrementally." Gorman collected stories of the myths and realities of famous inventions, pointing out that the telephone was not invented by Alexander Graham Bell, and that a light bulb existed before Thomas Edison invented it (he just found a way to more efficiently produce light). "The car industry epitomizes incremental innovations, from bikes to bikes with engines to cars," Gorman went on. "The television happened because teams of tinkerers and scientists around the world were working to build a radio for images, combining the technology of a wireless telegraph with the magic of a movie projector."

"We just need to forge ahead with our work and see where it leads us," Gorman concluded.

The men made their way back to Columbia. They had plans to return to Sing Sing in three days to draw blood from the subjects. They had wanted to return the next day, but Warden Denno changed their schedule, saying he didn't want the inmates to know exactly when they were coming. Sing Sing had a history of creative escapes, where prisoners broke out by fashioning dummies in their cells or by disguising themselves in guard uniforms. One inmate even sewed himself inside a mattress being removed from the prison. Under Denno's watch, no one had escaped. He intended to keep it that way.

Back in his office, Gorman sat down and took a deep breath. It had been a long day—and a wild one. With each step, the battle to defeat Rh seemed slightly more winnable, and a solution felt closer to his grasp, thanks to the bravery of the unlikely subjects at Sing Sing and the persistence of his friend and collaborator Vince Freda. Gorman's earlier doubts about staying in America had vanished. He hadn't made a name for himself—and he was far from wealthy—but he felt that his life was about to change.

CHAPTER NINE
Red-Blooded James

Even as the golden light of day faded to dusk, the Australian summer sun was scorching. James continued digging in his yard, sweat streaming down his face. Barb could see him from the kitchen window. Every weekend, as Barb did her cooking, needlepoint, and prepared her classwork for the week ahead, James dug up a stump around their home. There were thirty-two stumps in all, and James had committed to tackling one stump per week until there were no more.

"I'm not the sharpest knife in the drawer," James liked to say, "but I can get the job done."

James and Barb had been married for nearly six years. It was 1964, and James was twenty-eight years old. They had bought their starter home in Doonside, a suburb in western Sydney. James painted the house himself, built the fences, put in pathways, and did the landscaping— becoming something of a tree-removal specialist. He was fit and strong and didn't mind the hard labor. During the week, he sat behind a desk in his office at the railway, where he now had two people working under him. He spent most of his days finding out where the transit problems were and checking in with the railway's five branches, from mechanical to traffic, and writing up reports. One of his favorite parts of the job was visiting different stations, where he got to see kids stare in wonder at the giant steam engines. It transported him to his childhood: to the model trains that kept him company when he was sick and stuck inside and to the whistle of trains only blocks away, beckoning him back outside.

Brimming with energy, James sought out volunteer work that was physical. He built houses for the poor and offered to do home repairs for the elderly. He had helped start the Junee chapter of Apex, a young men's club, in 1956. When he moved to Sydney for work, he joined and built up the Apex chapter there. The club comprised mostly blue-collar laborers. In addition to building homes and providing meals to the elderly and poor, James set up information stands around town to raise money and recruit donors to his favorite cause—the Sydney blood bank. He attended Apex meetings every other Monday night, and had the highest number of service hours of anyone in the Sydney chapter. Barb became involved as a spouse and had the second-highest number of service hours herself. She raised money for Apex by selling her knits and needlepoint work.

When it was finally too dark to do any more yard work, James was called inside for dinner. Barb loved to see her husband devour whatever she cooked up. James boasted to friends: "Daughters of farmers are the best cooks." Barb had lived through difficult times in her childhood, with prolonged droughts that devastated the wheat crops. She had relished the bountiful times, when the family knew it would make it through the year.

Sitting down to rest and enjoy a glass of lemonade, James realized he and Barb had never really had a harsh word or bad day between them. From the start of their marriage, they pooled their income, never considering anything "his" or "hers." They had the household chores figured out: He did everything on the outside, and she took care of much on the inside, though James had discovered that he liked to shop for groceries and set the table. But some things never changed: James still left his clothes on the floor and couldn't cook to save his life.

The holidays were fast approaching, bringing Christmas and James's twenty-ninth birthday on December 27.

"Dad is doing his usual Santa Claus," James said. "He'll be gettin' on the train at four A.M. to roll into towns as Santa. Mom has freshened up his Santa suit." Reginald Harrison had become a beloved figure in Junee, where he was referred to either as "Mr. Junee" or "Fatty Harrison," a moniker he accepted with his typical good humor. He was stocky and rosy cheeked and took pride in what he called his "sturdy frame." He was as reliable and kind as anyone could be.

As Barb and James finished dinner, plaintive whines coming from the back door grew more urgent. James could see the darling faces of their new family members: pug dogs named Melinda and Monte. They'd bought them as puppies and were now breeding them.

Melinda and Monte loved weekends, when they were allowed inside for long stretches. Saturday was their favorite day—bath day. They were washed out back in a plastic kiddie pool and would then run dripping wet in tight and frenetic circles, their rear ends low to the ground like rabbits. After their circular sprints, they'd get to come inside for the day. The pugs would tear across the tile floor, get no traction, and slide their way to the living room.

"I'm quite happy with my lot," James said to Barb, taking the dishes to the kitchen and letting the pugs in for an evening visit. "As long as we are together and have a roof over our heads, I'm happy." Hank Williams, one of their favorites, was on the record player. James often quoted Williams: "If a song can't be written in twenty minutes, it ain't worth writing." Barb and James, being country music fans, had followed with amusement the news of the Beatles' tour in Australia and New Zealand. The Fab Four performed dozens of concerts in eight cities, and created a frenzy wherever they went, shutting down train stations and clogging streets. James preferred Johnny Cash to John Lennon any day of the week.

When James returned to the table, he could see Barb was lost in thought. She sometimes drifted like this, and he was pretty sure it was over the same worry. She was anxious that they might not be able to have children of their own. Before they were married, she had an ovarian cyst removed, leaving her with one working ovary. The doctor continued to monitor her for any underlying conditions.

James made a mental note to see whether he could get information from his friends at the Red Cross. He didn't want Barb to endure the kind of losses that he'd heard about at the blood bank.

The following week, James made his regular visit to 1 York Street. A white donor mobile was parked out front, the windows open for cross ventilation in the summer heat. He was surprised to find that Nurse Lizzie wasn't at the front desk. "She's just taking a lunch break," one of the nurses told him. "Or she's got her nose in a book."

Sure enough, just as James got himself situated in the donor chair, Nurse Lizzie appeared. She talked excitedly and showed him the book she was reading, *Blood Groups in Man*. "This was coauthored, *by a woman*," Lizzie beamed. "A woman from Australia named Ruth Sanger. This is the most important book out there on blood groups!"

James tried to share some of his news from work, telling her that the first double-decker trains had begun trial runs on the Sydney rail network. Lizzie, normally a rapt listener, was fixated on her book. James took one look at a photo of Ruth Sanger and said, "Not bad looking, now is she?"

Lizzie rolled her eyes and gave him a soft slug on the shoulder. She knew James was a red-blooded male, in every sense of the phrase.

"She graduated from the University of Sydney in 1938," Lizzie said of Ruth Sanger. Lizzie continued reading, noting that Sanger worked at the Red Cross transfusion service and went on to become one of the world's leading blood researchers. Lizzie attended to James's blood draw as she spoke. To study in England, Sanger had to sell her only asset, the family's piano. She traveled by ship in 1946. James could tell Lizzie was living vicariously through Sanger's adventures. Lizzie said that Sanger's PhD thesis was called "The multiplicity of blood group systems," and became the foundation for *Blood Groups in Man*.

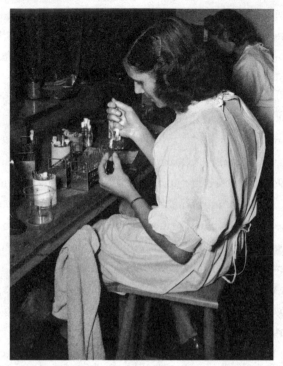

Ruth Sanger doing blood research and testing in New South Wales in the 1940s, before departing Australia to study in England.

"Look at this," she said, pointing to a letter written by Sanger's husband and coauthor, Robert Race: "Our work is primarily concerned with research into human blood groups, which is of the utmost importance in the practical problems of blood transfusion and certain blood diseases of the newborn."

James nodded, happy to have the distraction. He still had to look away every time a needle was near him.

"Ruth then became involved in this project to determine gene frequencies in the Rh system," Lizzie said, enthralled. "Remember, that's where you get the positive or negative factor in your blood typing. People are either Rhesus positive or Rhesus negative. Eighty-five percent of the population has Rhesus-positive blood type. So Ruth was doing work on Rh disease in the mums and babies in the early 1940s! Imagine that! She was apparently one of the researchers who found the relationship between the Rhesus factor and the incidence of these terrible miscarriages and deaths in newborns."

James knew there was no point in trying to say anything. When Lizzie got excited, whether over birds or blood typing, there was no interrupting.

Lizzie was surprised to learn that Sydney had started a program as early as 1943 to create a central blood bank for Rhesus-negative blood. "I didn't know anything about this," Lizzie said. "I have to look into it." She set the book down and reached for James's file. "You are Rh negative," she said. Then she flipped through pages filled with handwritten entries. She landed on something that puzzled her.

"Now this is kind of strange," she said, showing him his file. "You are *Rh-negative*. But you are testing positive for Rh-positive antibodies. Did we get something wrong?"

James looked down at his arm and held a small cotton swab over the dot of blood. He winked at Lizzie and said, "It proves, finally, that I'm special."

CHAPTER TEN
The Trials of Prison

In Sing Sing's sick bay, John Gorman and Vince Freda unpacked their cooler and the immunoglobulin—the purified blood serum—for another round of inmate injections and blood draws. They had been making regular visits to the notorious penitentiary for a year and a half and were now deep into their Rh trials.

The day felt like any other at Sing Sing. Prisoners were out in the yard playing basketball and softball, lifting weights and pitching horseshoes. Small groups of inmates in gray uniforms stood against walls, arguing over sports. There were the usual shouts of protest and melodramatic pleas for help. There was the tinny smell, the buzzing of metal doors, the clanking of keys, and the terse orders by guards. This had become the norm for Gorman and Freda, who were by now accustomed to the sights and sounds of the Big House.

The inmate who served as their bookkeeper—the accountant before Sing Sing—stood next to Gorman, recording in perfect columns the time and date, inmate information, and amounts of antibody or Rh-positive cells with the control and test groups. Another prisoner, inmate D. Maldonado, chatted with Freda. He struck Gorman and Freda as a particularly bright and capable guy who was in for a nonviolent offense. He had only a few months left to serve, and Gorman and Freda said they would try to get him a job at the Columbia Presbyterian hospital once he was released.

As the injections and blood draws progressed, the inmates relaxed and seemed to enjoy the banter, both with the doctors and among themselves. Gorman put the Vacutainers of collected blood in the cooler.

Bill Pollack of Ortho, who had provided the Rh-antibody serum, had emphasized that the researchers needed to make sure that the blood product was not denatured or compromised by being too warm or too cold.

The physicians thanked the prisoners one by one for their continued participation in the study. As usual, inmate J. Fox—who was in for robbery—once again told Gorman: "Don't do the crime if you can't do the time." Gorman and Freda told the guys that they would see them "soon."

"See ya," Freda said. One of the inmates was still talking to Gorman, and Freda had to gently pull him away.

In the next instant, though, everything went silent. No one moved.

A shout came from outside the room: "Riot!"

The shout grew louder: "Riot!"

A sea of gray uniforms moved in formation just outside the sick bay. Guards drew weapons.

"They got him!" someone shouted. "This is going to be ugly."

For Gorman and Freda, the next minute was a blur. Guards pushed the two doctors out of the sick ward and into a closed passageway. Gorman, heart racing, clutching the cooler, stole a glance back. The inmates had formed a line of defense. He thought: *They were protecting us.*

Another yell echoed through the building: "Stabbing! Man down." Next came the sounds of a stampede.

Sirens wailed and heavy boots moved in fast formation. War had erupted inside Sing Sing.

Gorman and Freda were rushed through the halls, out several doors, and finally escorted past the two iron gates. The guards turned and disappeared back inside the prison. Visibly shaken, Gorman and Freda ran to their car. A woman named Nancy Treacy, whom Gorman and Freda had hired as a technician to help with the trial—though she was not allowed inside the prison—was surprised to see them. She had remained in the parked car just outside the prison gates. Gorman and Freda, out of breath, jumped in.

"Let's get out of here!" Gorman said. "There was a stabbing."

"There's a riot!" Freda said.

Treacy sped off. There would be no stops for lunch and martinis today. Gorman and Freda sat in stunned silence. Finally, Gorman said, "That came out of nowhere. Or did I miss something?" Gorman rifled through the many warnings he'd been given about Sing Sing. Even Freda had told him: "Don't get too comfortable. They're in here for a reason." A guard who had picked up on Gorman's trusting nature told him: "One of your guys may be so perfectly respectful. Then you find out that he cut his mother's head off or pushed a kid out a window." Until now, Gorman hadn't believed the warnings. The men he dealt with in the trial were polite and respectful.

Gorman mulled over the Sing Sing he thought he knew versus the Sing Sing he'd seen that day. He had been told that this was a place where gang rapes went unreported, where fights and riots broke out over changed family day schedules, food that was too hot, too cold, too spicy, not spicy enough. But he had seen a prison that was orderly, even friendly. "It's very clean and civilized," Gorman had told his girlfriend, Carol, after a recent visit.

Taking in the snow-dusted landscape outside the car window on the way back to Columbia, Gorman finally concluded that Sing Sing was a place of contrasts: where slugger Babe Ruth once blasted a home run over the yard wall in a game against the prison team, and where brutal punishments were doled out. There was a fascination and a revulsion to life behind bars, to this world of compliance and defiance. There was betterment and punishment, and the balance of power was challenged every day. For Gorman, it was a place where supposedly bad men were trying to do something good. He was certain that when the riot started, these lawbreakers in the sick bay were going to protect him.

Gorman could see that Freda was also processing the events. He and his wife, Carol, had two young children now, and a third baby was on the way. Yet despite the dangerous prison scare, both Gorman and Freda knew there was no turning back. The trials were showing too much promise.

The first phase of the trials—involving the nine inmates—had supported Gorman's theory that the introduction of passive antibodies would prevent the creation of active antibodies. None of the four men given the passive Rh antibodies before the injection of Rh-positive cells had become actively immunized. But four of the five who had not received the prophylactic had become actively immunized. The objective of the trial, of course, was to see whether the doctors could *prevent* immunization—or sensitization—through the passive antibodies. Initiation of immunity to Rh was the pernicious event that could threaten the future of the Rh-negative mother and her unborn Rh-positive child. If Gorman and Freda could prevent sensitization in male volunteers, they would begin testing in women.

Phase two of the Sing Sing trials involved twenty-seven inmates. Gorman and Freda, working closely with Bill Pollack, had kept to the same concentration—or titer—of the antibody serum. So far, the phase one successes in New York had not been duplicated by the team in Liverpool. Using volunteer policemen instead of inmates, the Liverpool group had run into trouble with their tests using a different Rh antibody. The British researchers were relying on the 19S Rh antibody instead of the 7S Rh antibody, as Gorman and Freda used. (Human antibodies are classified into five types. The 7S antibody—also known as the IgG isotype—is the antibody most people think of when they talk about antibodies. It is the later-appearing antibody built by immunization.) It turned out that the passive 19S antibody used by the Brits *enhanced* the immune response. It provoked an even stronger immune reaction and thus was the opposite of what they were trying to achieve, and aroused fears that the whole program there could be derailed.

Once Gorman and Freda arrived back at Freda's tiny research lab at Columbia, they shook off the unsettling events of the day. They would return to the prison in three days, assuming order was restored after the riot. Nancy Treacy went to work in Freda's lab in the Rh clinic. She was meticulous and would first do a Coombs test to see whether the latest samples contained Rh antibodies. To do this, she would put the plasma in a test tube, add a Rh-positive reagent red cells, and then add antihuman (rabbit or goat) IgG antibody. If agglutination occurred when the plasma was mixed with the agent, antibodies were present. The test had been developed by immunologist Robin Coombs (though it had been described decades earlier by an Italian researcher), who was among a group of renowned immunologists who came to prominence in Britain after World War II. The test was done by diluting a patient's plasma until there was less and less Rh antibody until, finally, the antibodies could no longer be detected. This would give Treacy the titer count she was looking for. It was all done with a manual pipette to transfer a measured amount of liquid into a row of test tubes.

Soon, the doctors got the green light to return to Sing Sing, and they resumed their trips up the Hudson River, albeit with the firsthand knowledge that the prison was a place of both routines and unpredictability. Over a few months, as Gorman and Freda waited for more of their results to come in, data from similar trials elsewhere began to surface.

The Liverpool team was now having improved results, after Pollack shared some of the Ortho gamma globulin using the 7S antibody. The Chown and Zipursky team in Canada was also advancing, and individual doctors and researchers were weighing in with their findings. The risky trial in St. Louis—risky because pregnant women were receiving whole blood that hadn't been fractionated—was showing promise.

It took more than two months for the results of the phase two Sing Sing trials to be tested and retested. Gorman and Freda met in Freda's lab to review results. It wasn't lost on Gorman that only a handful of years earlier, Freda had walked into the blood bank and asked for every record available on women with Rh disease. They had started this chase by looking for clues on hundreds of 3x5 cards. Now they were finding answers from Sing Sing prisoners.

Gorman and Freda studied the results from the twenty-seven men. For a moment, Gorman thought Freda was teary-eyed.

Finally, Gorman said it: "The results are beautiful."

The twenty-seven men had each been given two injections of Rh-positive cells at six-month intervals. Although active immunity was stimulated in eight of the thirteen controls, none of the fourteen men given 5 milliliters Rh-immune globulin seventy-two hours after the first injection and forty-eight hours after the second injection became immunized.

Gorman and Freda went over the results again, line by line. The Sing Sing trials had shown that Rh immunoglobulin in adequate dosage would provide protection against sensitization by an intense antigenic stimulus much greater than the stimulus of the average Rh-positive pregnancy. More trials would be needed, but this was a victory. A victory that had started with a passage in a textbook. Gorman and Freda were on to something revolutionary.

Gorman looked at his watch, patted Freda on the shoulder, and apologized that he had to hustle back to his office. He was meeting his girlfriend, Carol, for dinner. Before he met her, he wanted to dash off a letter to his parents. Back at his desk, he began: "Vince Freda and I have beautiful results from Sing Sing . . ."

Gorman left his office walking on air. He was nothing if not a believer in basic research, in simple ideas that make a big difference. To him, problems were tractable. Nobel Prizes were awarded for esoteric work; out of a simple desire for knowledge came breakthroughs. What couldn't be predicted was the eventual value of newfound knowledge. Could lives be saved by a simple adjustment to the immune system, by giving the body something it already had? The thinking, at least for Gorman, was based on the intelligence of the immune system: If it has enough of a certain antibody, it won't make more. The body had hundreds of control systems regulating everything from hemoglobin to hormones. Gorman believed that the passive antibodies wouldn't harm the baby because of dosage levels. Using a minute amount of the antibodies would coat the baby's Rh-positive cells, but not in a way that would cause anemia.

Driving to pick up Carol, Gorman knew that he still had a long and winding road ahead. Trials could come undone at any time. They would need more trials, and more antibodies. They would need new funding and bigger trials. This felt urgent, though research could be plodding.

While taking in the tapestry of lights in Manhattan, Gorman believed more strongly than ever that he had been right in coming to America. This was a place where anything was possible, a place that felt much more egalitarian than Australia, where the more rigid British class system was very much intact. He was thirty-four years old, had finished his residency, ending his long years of medical training, and now was involved in a promising trial that just might lead to a break-through. His salary had jumped to a more comfortable $15,000 a year.

Arriving at the restaurant, he wondered aloud: "Why would anyone ever want to live anywhere but Manhattan?" Things were falling into place. He just needed one other thing to become conclusive in his life: Carol. Over the months, as his research into Rh had progressed in fits and starts, so had their relationship.

Just as Carol had to learn to navigate John's quiddities and preoccupations, John had done his best to navigate Carol's personality. He was no longer the shy, stammering young doctor who loved medicine but disliked patients. He had arrived at Columbia an unknown, and had his ideas discounted and dismissed. But time was advancing. His career was advancing. He wanted Carol to be his wife. The research and clinical trial phase of the relationship was over. Besides, he knew that Carol had a history of ditching more than one fiancé at the altar or in the days or weeks leading up to the wedding. He had heard stories of how she would tearfully cancel at the last minute, certain she was making the wrong decision. So, at dinner that night, when Carol again seemed to be wavering on the idea of marrying, John wasn't having it. He stopped eating, set his napkin on the table, pointed to the clock on the wall and said, "Here's the deal. The clock is ticking. I'm going to Australia for two weeks. When I come back, I need an answer." Carol was startled, but promised an answer.

Less than a month later, John and Carol were married in the Fifth Avenue Presbyterian Church in New York. John wasn't about to risk a long engagement. Even on such short notice, the chapel was packed; Vince and Carol Freda served as best man and maid of honor. John wore a black suit, white shirt, and silver tie, and had a white flower in his lapel. Carol wore a sleeveless brocade dress, red lipstick, and her hair swept back in a French twist.

They flew to Australia for their honeymoon, where the newlyweds were greeted by the Gorman clan and spent most of their time in the beach town of Barwon Heads, where John's family had a cottage. Carol quickly bonded with John's father, John Sextus Gorman, who went by Jack, and joined him on long walks on the beach. John's mother, Jean Elma Doris Grant, who went by Doris, and Carol found common ground in medicine, and in their love for John. Carol enjoyed hearing stories from the Gorman women. One of John's cousins told Carol that she'd recently spotted a deadly snake out back, quickly set her baby in a basket, grabbed a rifle, and shot the snake—all with the casual ease of someone retrieving the mail.

As the honeymoon in Australia wound down, Carol was excited to return to New York. The Fredas were going to throw a party for them, and both John and Carol were looking forward to settling in to married life. But while Carol and John were packing the night before their scheduled departure, Carol sensed something was up.

"We are leaving tomorrow, right?" Carol asked.

"Yes," John replied.

"To go home," she continued.

John looked at her sheepishly. "Well, not exactly," he said.

"*Not exactly*? What does that mean? Where are we going then?"

After a pause that seemed to last forever, John said, "New Guinea."

Carol, the daughter of a Calvinist minister from Grand Rapids, Michigan, who had never been out of the U.S. until her honeymoon, was speechless. Finally, she said, "Where is New Guinea? Why in the world are we going to *New Guinea*?"

"You couldn't go to a more beautiful place than New Guinea," John offered. He didn't tell her that on an earlier trip there, he had been bitten by a centipede while sleeping and thought he was going to die, or that the pilots on the route to New Guinea were cowboys who loved to fly as low as possible over deserted beaches. He certainly didn't tell her that Nelson Rockefeller's son, Michael Rockefeller, had died there, and was either eaten by alligators or tribesmen.

Carol wasn't moved by the "beautiful place" comment. John, who never had a gift of timing when it came to women, knew he needed to fess up.

"We are going to study glucose-6-phosphate dehydrogenase deficiency and its connection to malaria," he said. "In the mountains of New Guinea, there is no malaria, but on the coast it's rampant, so we are going to compare the blood of people in the highlands to those on the coast."

He added, "You can do the blood draws. You're so good with everyone."

Carol could not believe her ears. "You didn't think of telling me we were going to New Guinea on our honeymoon?" She searched her mind for any information she had on New Guinea. Finally, she said, "Isn't New Guinea where they eat people?"

John replied, "They only eat dead people." He didn't think that perhaps this wasn't the most reassuring answer to give to his new bride.

The next day, they boarded a DC-3 with a handful of passengers to fly to New Guinea. They landed in a field in the center of the town of Garoka, where they were whisked away in jeeps through the thick jungle. The driver kept looking back at Carol. In broken English, he said, "She go there, too?" John nodded. He then looked at Carol, as if seeing her for the first time, and told her, "I think what you're wearing is maybe too cute." Carol just shook her head. The jeep was barreling along the rugged dirt road. They had passed the point of no return.

After some time climbing into the hills, they arrived in a tribal center. As soon as they were out of the jeep, Carol was swarmed by tribespeople. Everyone wanted to touch her hair, as no one had ever seen a blonde before. Carol was stunned by something else, too: No one wore a shred of clothing, except the chief, who had a loincloth. The chief appeared bewitched by Carol and introduced her to his nine wives. One of her first tasks would be to draw blood from the chief's forty children.

Carol looked around and spotted John energetically setting up his lab equipment. He had Vacutainers, alcohol swabs, and a test he had developed himself in the lab at Columbia to take into the field. If the gene for the glucose-6-phosphate dehydrogenase deficiency existed, the blood sample turned blue, thanks to the chemicals that John had concocted in the lab. Carol couldn't help but smile. Life with John would certainly not be boring. Even in the few years she had known him, she had seen him grow into his ambition. He was becoming the man he set out to be in America. A childhood friend from Bendigo had recently visited and marveled: "You're not the shy John Gorman I remember!"

John was proud of how Carol was handling herself. He also felt like he was in his element here, an unlikely swashbuckler on an incredible adventure in a land that few had explored. He was a far cry from the bashful tinkerer who had hung out in his workshop during his childhood, or the reticent doctor who had hid in the research room to avoid patients. Now he found himself in the cells of Sing Sing, the jungles of New Guinea, and wherever his research took him.

John had finally learned to embrace the unexpected. But the unexpected was about to embrace him with one of his biggest tests yet.

CHAPTER ELEVEN
A Daring Delivery

On their drive to the airport, John Gorman noticed that Vince Freda was quiet and even more fidgety than usual. Gorman understood why: The two men were embarking on a secret, audacious mission—not without risks—and were about to bend a number of rules. But Gorman was steadfastly confident that their surreptitious efforts were for the greater good—and just might save lives.

He had a deeply personal motive, too.

In the car, Freda kept his eyes glued to a small Styrofoam container on the floor of the passenger seat, wedged between his feet. Gorman, making small talk, wondered aloud whether Harlem River Drive or I-95 would be the fastest route to Idlewild—forgetting for a moment that the New York airport had been renamed John F. Kennedy International a year earlier, following the assassination of the nation's thirty-fifth president.

The tightly sealed container at Freda's feet was being shipped from JFK to Heathrow Airport in London, England. The package contained a carefully packed vial of the Ortho-produced Rh antibody. If everything went according to plan, it would be used on a pregnant woman for the first time ever, having until now only been tested on men at Sing Sing. That woman was none other than Gorman's twenty-three-year-old sister-in-law, Kath Gorman, who was married to his younger brother Frank. Kath was Rh negative, and Frank was Rh positive. They had been told that this first baby, if Rh positive like Frank, would probably be fine but would "sensitize" Kath—activating her antibodies to the Rh antigen—in a way that could harm or kill her future children. Gorman knew that Kath needed the Rh serum right after childbirth, or it could be too late. He didn't have time to wait for a labyrinth of follow-up trials—this was his family, after all. Furthermore, he believed to his core that he had found a life-changing treatment to Rh that needed to get out in the world as soon as possible. To him, the benefits of today's below-the-radar mission far exceeded any potential risk or harm.

Gorman and Freda had confided their plan to only a few—aware that they were shipping an experimental biological product out of the country to be used by doctors who were not approved to administer the treatment. Only Gorman and Freda were authorized to inject the medicine, and only in the United States. They had not even shared their decision with Bill Pollack at Ortho.

The idea for the intervention had come from Gorman's father in Australia, who was closely following his son's Rh trials at Columbia. He had been thrilled to read John's most recent letter about the "beautiful" results of the second phase of the Sing Sing trials. So, when the senior Gorman learned that Frank and Kath were expecting their first child in England, he asked about their blood types. Upon learning of the blood incompatibility, his letters to Frank grew increasingly urgent, telling him: "You've got to do something about this." He was a general practitioner in Bendigo and spent a good amount of time in obstetrics. He was all too familiar with Rh disease.

Gorman and Freda arrived at JFK late, having been slowed by traffic. They rushed through the airport terminal, taking one wrong turn after the other until they found the customs and freight area. Gorman quickly filled out the paperwork. Under the question about contents, Gorman paused before writing "HUMAN SERUM." Freda paced nearby, keeping an eye on the container. In the end, it was his friend's confidence that convinced him this was the right thing to do, despite the rules they were surely breaking. Gorman was so sure of the safety of the Rh treatment that he was willing to use it on his own family. To Freda, there couldn't be a greater endorsement. But as the container with the Rh vial, packed in dry ice, was taken away for shipping, Freda was again consumed with worries: *Where would it be stored? Would the medical staff in England follow the protocols as dictated by Gorman? Would someone step in to block the injection? Would he and Gorman land themselves in legal or medical trouble?* The container was set atop a pile of boxes, and then hauled away. It was now out of their hands, and out of their control. *This is crazy*, Freda thought. The Rh treatment had never been used clinically—anywhere.

Gorman and Freda drove back to the city, saying very little. Hours of discussion had already gone into getting to this point. Now they would hope for the best.

Back at Columbia, Freda headed to the hospital and Gorman to the blood bank. Freda had babies to deliver and was preparing for their trials at the Columbia Rh clinic. This phase would treat Rh-incompatible first pregnancies and subsequent deliveries in women who had not already developed antibodies to the Rh antigen. Coincidentally, the researchers in Liverpool had reported they were also ready to start their trials involving pregnant women, having had more success after switching to the antibody formula that Pollack had shared. Gorman returned to his office, dealt with urgent calls, and made note of the time. The vial was well on its way to England.

A few hours later, at a flat in the London suburb of Finchley Road, Frank and Kath Gorman rang up Heathrow to check the status of their package. They were told the plane was on time and would arrive that night. Kath was due in two weeks, giving them plenty of time to confirm plans and go over details again with her own doctors.

Kath and Frank decided to head to Heathrow but stop for dinner along the way. They got into their much-loved secondhand Mercedes— bought for £50—and took off in the direction of Heathrow, about an hour away. Even at the end of her pregnancy, Kath was petite, though she declared herself "enormous." She had dark hair, brown eyes, a quick mind, and a clever sense of humor. She was a nurse when she met Frank Gorman, who was an ophthalmologist. They were both in Derby in western Australia working for the Royal Flying Doctor Service, which provided emergency and basic health services to those living in rural and remote areas of the country. Kath later worked as a pediatric nurse, a job that suited her pragmatic but cheerful disposition. She loved children and wanted a big family of her own.

After getting a bite to eat, they arrived at Heathrow and asked for directions to customs and shipping.

"I'm not feeling good," Kath told Frank as they walked.

"Probably indigestion," Frank said, walking ahead of her.

"No, I'm getting these pains in my stomach, where it feels really hard," Kath said.

Frank paused. "Does the pain stop when you change positions, from sitting to standing?"

"No, it's just these hard waves," Kath said.

Frank looked at her closely and said: "You silly idiot, you're in labor." Then he said, "Can you make it?"

Kath had never been pregnant before but assured him she would be fine. She focused on her breathing. Looking around the grimy airport, she wondered what she would do if she had to deliver here. When they finally found the freight area, they had to wait for what felt like an eternity. Frank chatted away like nothing was happening while Kath dealt with contractions. Finally, paperwork signed, Frank paid the customs fee, grumbling about the cost—wondering aloud how a sum was placed on human serum—and handed Kath the container.

She laughed. The container looked like a bowl she'd make a cake in. It was white with green spots and had a flat lid. Inside, though, were very different ingredients: dry ice and a vial of antibodies. The two returned to the parking garage, and Kath eased herself back into the small car. She held the container upright, as if the liquid inside was at risk of spilling out.

"Here we thought we had all the time in the world," Kath said, breathing through the contractions. "After months of back and forth, we almost missed this."

Back home, they packed a bag for the hospital, and got back in the car. Kath and Frank had talked early on in her pregnancy with their prenatal doctor about the Rh blood incompatibility. The doctor had told them matter of factly that he had "nothing to offer" them. There was no treatment for Rh disease. The Rh trials on the policemen in Liverpool—only four hours away from where they lived in Finchley Road—had been inconsistent until recently. After considerable pressure, Kath's doctor had at least agreed to talk with her brother-in-law in New York. John Gorman then took over, explaining the treatment and the results of the Sing Sing trial. He followed up by sending the doctor the supporting paperwork and trial data. A pathologist was then brought in to consult with Kath's doctor on the case. Almost all the back and forth was done without involving Kath—who protested, "I'm the guinea pig here!" But she knew that once the Gorman men got involved with anything medical, there was no getting a word in.

She had learned early in her courtship with Frank that the Gormans were a close-knit—and talented—clan. John was the firstborn, followed by Frank (born Richard Francis Gorman), Jocelyn, and Jeanne. Kath loved hearing Gorman stories, first of their childhood in the city of Rochester, and then in the gold mining town of Bendigo. One story had especially captivated Kath. Now in the car—in labor with a human blood serum on her lap—seemed like a good time for a distraction.

Frank was happy to oblige, launching into his story of "the summer of 1937," when he was five and John was six. The polio epidemic had hit Australia hard, creating fear and widespread panic among families and doctors. The unpredictable and incurable virus swept through towns in the hot summer months. Houses were fumigated, families ostracized, and people quarantined. Hospitalized children were put into body splints and iron lungs. The viral disease mostly targeted children, and the worst cases caused paralysis and death. John Gorman Sr. became spooked when one of his neighbor's children, a girl named Helen who was close in age to John, contracted the virus. The senior Gorman hastily arranged to get his boys out of the county and into New South Wales, where his brother Dick lived—and where there were no reported cases of polio. The problem was, no children were being allowed in. Police were stationed on every bridge going into the Murray River area of New South Wales.

To the Gorman boys, the two-hour road trip was a grand adventure. They rode in the back of Uncle Dick's car, playing games and eating sandwiches. Shortly before crossing the Murray River on the Swan Hill Bridge, Uncle Dick—not one to be disobeyed—ordered the boys to get as flat as possible on the floor of the back seat. He threw a blanket over them and told them not to say a word until he removed the blanket. The boys didn't dare move a hair. They barely breathed as they listened to Uncle Dick talk casually with the police officer before being waved through.

Uncle Dick's sheep station in New South Wales was spread over fifty thousand acres and was split evenly with another Gorman brother, Brendan. There were ten miles of dirt roads leading to the front gate, which was twenty-three miles from Robinvale and had fifteen miles of gorgeous frontage on the winding Murray River. Frank and John spent three months there, working long hours at the ranch, shearing sheep, milking cows, and taking care of the animals. But they also had time to fish with spinners, ride ponies, swim in the crystal-clear river, and sleep outside on the ranch's wraparound veranda. There was no electricity, so kerosene lamps provided the only light at night. All around them at the ranch were hundreds of emu and kangaroo. Their favorite part of their stay was when they were put in charge of the care of an orphaned joey—a baby kangaroo. They fed it milk from a baby's bottle and watched it grow. At the end of their stay at the ranch, they watched with tears streaming down their cheeks as the joey hopped the fence and took off without so much as a look back.

Frank, who had been lost in the story with Kath, checked his watch. They still had more than ten minutes to go. He asked Kath, "Did you know that Dr. Jonas Salk, who invented the polio vaccine, tested it out on himself and his family?" Kath understood what he was getting at. She suspected that Frank had worries about treating her with the Rh serum, but he hadn't shared them. Frank and Kath both had heard John talk about how Salk's work on the polio vaccine had been yet another confirmation of the immunosuppressive power of passive antibodies.

John also talked to Frank about similarities in the race among researchers to be first. Salk was the first to market with the polio vaccine, but close behind was another researcher, Albert Sabin, who separately developed an oral polio vaccine. The men had been seeking to eradicate the same thing, with one building on the other, much like the progression of the teams at Columbia and Liverpool.

Frank told Kath in the car, "John left Australia for America at around the same time Salk's vaccine was approved for treatment in 1955."

Kath, still trying to distract herself from the increasingly intense contractions, listened with interest but didn't find Frank's reference to scientists who self-experimented particularly reassuring. As a nurse, she had been around doctors and hospitals for years, and knew that even the most vigorous trials with heralded success could still have failures.

When Salk's vaccine went into a nationwide testing program suddenly, about two hundred cases of the disease were caused by the vaccine and eleven people died. It was discovered that one poorly made batch caused the problem. She remembered hearing of an awful case in Australia—known as the Bundaberg disaster—which involved the death of a dozen children after receiving inoculations of diphtheria toxin-antitoxin. The vial used to inoculate the children was contaminated. There was also the risk, John had acknowledged, that the Rh-positive antibodies might "sensitize" Kath when she may not have been sensitized otherwise, thus harming any future babies. She didn't yet know the blood type of her baby. She might not even need the injection.

But her father-in-law had been unrelenting in his push to get the treatment to Kath, and Frank, wholly unconcerned for the first few months, had finally agreed, saying, "Okay, we all have faith in John." Kath would get the injection after she delivered, so at least there was no threat to the baby if something went wrong. Finally arriving at the hospital, Kath was "pretty certain" the Rh treatment wasn't going to harm her, but it was impossible to completely ignore the potential risks, no matter how seemingly remote.

Already in labor, Kath was admitted and sent to delivery, though the doctors said she would probably not deliver until the morning. Frank went home to sleep and said he'd return in the morning. Kath struggled through the night. This was not an easy delivery. Early in the morning, things took a turn for the worse, and the doctors grew concerned. The baby's head had moved up against Kath's pelvic bone and wasn't shifting. There was talk of a C-section. An attending obstetrician said he would try to manually rotate the baby internally. It worked, but came with excruciating pain to Kath and caused profuse bleeding.

Outside Kath's room, one of the doctors on call was unaware of the Rh vial and the months of back and forth between Kath's doctor and the Gorman team in New York. Fortunately, the pathologist who had been briefed on the situation was nearby and filled the on-call doctor in on the experimental treatment, the Sing Sing trials, and the trials in nearby Liverpool. The doctor studied the files and letters. He wasn't at all convinced. He picked up the phone to call the researchers in Liverpool.

Time was running out. Kath's baby was now in position to move down the birth canal. Frank arrived at the hospital to find the pathologist and an unfamiliar doctor talking with someone from the University of Liverpool. He heard the doctor say that if the Liverpool researchers wouldn't confirm it, he wouldn't go ahead with the injection.

"We've got Gorman's sister or maybe sister-in-law here, and we've got this Rh treatment from America," the doctor said. There was a long pause. Frank imagined that the team from Liverpool—Cyril Clarke, Ronnie Finn, Richard McConnell—was hearing of this for the first time. He could imagine their surprise: Liverpool followed every development at Columbia, as Columbia devoured any news from Liverpool. Frank approached the desk, ready to intervene.

Finally, the doctor nodded, scribbled notes, and said, "Okay, yes, yes," and hung up.

"What did they say?" Frank asked nervously.

"They didn't sound happy," the doctor said, making Frank's heart sink. "But they said, 'Yes, give it to her.' They want me to send her blood samples from before and after the injection."

Within minutes, the cry of a newborn was heard through the halls. Kath and Frank had a baby boy, Kieron Francis Gorman. It was January 31, 1964. He was two weeks early but healthy and rosy cheeked, weighing in at eight pounds, eleven ounces. He had reddish hair, hazel eyes, and was "a Gorman to look at," Kath declared.

The technicians stepped in to draw blood from Kath and baby Kieron. The results came back quickly. Kieron's blood type was Rh positive, like his father—and incompatible with his mother. A sample of Kath's blood was taken. Through the Kleihauer–Betke test, the doctors were able to measure the amount of fetal blood that had gotten into Kath's bloodstream. Kath had a huge amount of Kieron's Rh-positive blood in her system, not surprising given the struggles of her delivery. The vial marked human serum, which started its journey in New York, was now needed.

After double-checking the blood results, the doctor arrived in Kath's room holding the Rh vial, which was still sealed with the rubber membrane. Frank signed more papers, again taking full responsibility for the experimental treatment. The doctor told Kath to roll on her side and lift her gown to expose her backside. As the needle went into her gluteus muscle, Kath made a comment that made everyone laugh: "Imagine this: I'm an *Australian* patient given an *American* injection in an *English* hospital!"

After what Kath had already been through, she barely noticed the shot. She was monitored closely through the night, with a nurse arriving hourly to tell her to roll over so she could check for a rash. In the middle of the night, Kath began to sweat profusely and soaked her gown and sheets. But by morning, she was fine again, and her temperature had regulated.

Frank called New York to connect with John, who told him not to worry. Night sweats had been reported by some of the inmates at Sing Sing, and the problem would likely not persist for more than one night.

A few days later, Kath and Kieron went home. After the difficult delivery, Kath was moving slowly, but she was entirely devoted to her big baby boy, who seemed to her as intelligent and insistent as a Gorman should be.

Back in New York, John soon received a cable from Frank, who said their "well-timed gamble" was a success. John sat back and smiled. He had his first nephew. He folded the cable and tucked it in the top drawer of his desk. Despite his brother's glowing report, John knew that the success of the gamble wouldn't be known until Kath had another baby, and then another—and all were free of Rh disease. The victory would come when John had a gaggle of nephews and nieces—lives that would likely not have made it into the world without a rule-breaking transcontinental intervention.

CHAPTER TWELVE
A Revolution in Medicine

With all eyes on him, John Gorman removed his reading glasses from his breast pocket and headed toward the dais of the grand auditorium hall. It was August 1966, and hundreds of scientists, doctors, researchers, and nurses had poured into the sandstone buildings of the University of Sydney for the Eleventh Congress of the International Society of Blood Transfusion. The chair of the meeting was none other than Philip Levine, who discovered the mechanism of Rh disease. In the weeks leading up to the conference, there had been persistent rumors about the announcement of a major medical breakthrough of some kind, so many journalists and industry insiders were also on hand in anticipation of something big.

For Gorman, who had risen to the directorship of Columbia Presbyterian Hospital's blood bank, the moment was especially satisfying, given that the medical establishment had so thoroughly dismissed his ideas about combatting Rh disease. Now those ideas were front and center at a conference, which had attracted some of the top Rh researchers in the world.

Gorman, there with Vince Freda, was happy to be back in Australia. He was staying in the beautiful coastal suburb of Manly and enjoyed driving in and out of central Sydney and watching the construction of the dramatic "shells" of the Sydney Opera House. The building, long delayed and over budget, was finally taking shape. Ronnie Finn had arrived in Australia from Liverpool, as had noted blood researcher Alvin Zipursky, who ran the anti-Rh trial program in Canada. Many of the speakers and delegates were being housed in the University of Sydney dorms. Sydney hadn't hosted many international conferences before and had to plan the event around when university classes let out.

The conference had begun with various breakout sessions, including a discussion on the world's first successful intrauterine fetal blood transfusion by Bill Liley in New Zealand, and its implication for Rh disease. Gorman had listened attentively as a research scientist went through his presentation using a Kodak Carousel slide projector. Suddenly, when the slides began to inexplicably shake, the scientist quipped: "The slides may be shaky, but my presentation is rock solid." Gorman commended the presenter for his deft handling of the situation.

But the show that everyone had come for was in the main hall, where Gorman was preparing to speak to the delegates and attendees. He had been preceded to the center stage by an impressive lineup of researchers whom he greatly admired.

First off had been Alvin Zipursky, who was tall, lanky, energetic, and beloved by patients who knew him as "Zip." Zipursky began by talking about what had motivated him to start the Rh prevention trials in Canada years earlier. He was working as a pediatric hematologist—looking at blood disorders in children—and serving as director of the Red Cross blood transfusion service when he first heard about the potentially breakthrough research around Rh disease coming out of Columbia and Liverpool. He considered Rh one of the most devastating and dramatic diseases, "a Shakespearean tragedy" in which a mother's body unknowingly turns against her unborn child.

With excitement in his voice, he told the conference crowd that the premise for the treatment of Rh disease astounded him.

"Here was a dramatic solution, a paradox really, where the same agent that causes Rh disease and can kill babies in the womb is the very medicine to stop this," he said. "I thought, 'We must create our own Rh prevention program in Canada!'"

Zipursky had played a significant role in the understanding of Rh disease. In 1959, he caused a stir with his experiments on transplacental bleeds. His research revealed that small amounts of a baby's blood cross into the mother's circulation throughout pregnancy, and not just at delivery as was commonly believed. His paper about Rh transplacental bleeds was published in the *Lancet* and read with excitement by Ronnie Finn, Gorman, Freda, and others. Before Zipursky, the prevailing theory had been that the bleeds from baby to mother occurred only through trauma to the abdomen during gestation or, primarily, at delivery. Because of his findings, Zipursky now argued that the anti-Rh antibodies should be given *during* pregnancy, in contrast to the post-delivery protocol established by Gorman and Freda.

"So, after reading about the trials in New York and Liverpool, I set out to make my own Rh immune globulin, just as they had in Liverpool and in New York," Zipursky said. Winnipeg—Canada—became the third group in the world doing Rh disease prevention. Zipursky said he went to Dr. Bruce Chown, founder and director of Winnipeg's Rh laboratory and asked for the names of four women studied by the lab whose blood had high levels of Rh antibodies. He wanted to create a donor pool from women who had lost babies to Rh disease.

"I then set out into some of Winnipeg's poorest neighborhoods," he told the rapt audience. "I went to this house near the railroad tracks, walked up the stairs, and knocked on the door. There I was asking this woman who had suffered greatly: 'Will you agree to donate blood once a week?'" With tears in his eyes, Zipursky said, "One woman, Mary, had been pregnant eight times. Only her first baby was healthy and lived. Her second baby, Gerry, died a day after birth. Her third son was stillborn. Then came a miscarriage, and another. After her eighth, she decided no more dead babies."

The delegates were hanging on Zipursky's every word. "When I stood there at Mary's door and asked for help, she didn't hesitate. She said, 'Sign me up. I don't want this to happen to other women.' Mary is now a part of a group of four women who call themselves 'The Rh Ladies of Winnipeg.' I see them every Thursday morning."

Zipursky told the crowd that he obtained gamma globulin with Rh antibodies from the University of Toronto's Connaught Laboratories. "I flew to Toronto carrying a cooler full of the Rh Ladies' blood and came back with the first vial of gamma globulin, which I have on my desk. We began a trial with Rh-negative pregnant women."

Then, pausing for dramatic effect, Zipursky proclaimed: "Our findings show that the treatment is entirely effective in stopping Rh disease."

Applause reverberated through the hall. But that was only the beginning.

Next on stage was Ronnie Finn from Liverpool, who apologized that Cyril Clarke was unable to attend. Finn was hardworking and modest and—as a practicing Jew—often told people that he became a doctor to "give back some of what the Holocaust took away." Finn, nodding to Zipursky just off the stage, said he had been inspired in his own studies of Rh because of Zipursky's fetal bleed report published in the *Lancet*. After reading Zipursky's study, Finn focused on using the Kleihauer-Betke test to monitor the blood cells of Rh-negative mothers during pregnancy and after delivery. His research led him to suggest that if an Rh-negative mother were given anti-Rh antibody soon enough, any fetal red blood cells in her circulation would be inactivated before her immune system could become sensitized to the Rh antigen.

Finn briefed the gathered on the progress of the studies in Liverpool, which had expanded from the volunteer policemen to a trial begun a year earlier on Rh-negative mothers. Finn said that under Cyril Clarke's direction, the Liverpool researchers had proceeded cautiously, aware that they were moving from male volunteers to pregnant women, where "you don't make mistakes."

"Only mothers whose Kleihauer–Betke fetal cell–screening tests were positive—with fetal cells showing up in the maternal blood—were admitted to the trial," Finn said. These were mothers who were in their first pregnancies and were at especially high risk of becoming sensitized to the Rh factor. "We have very good evidence from our new trials. What we see is that when such high-risk Rh-negative mothers are treated by anti-Rh (passive antibodies), no sensitizations occur."

It was yet another revelation for the crowd. Day was turning into night, but no one made a move to leave. Gorman had listened to his colleagues with interest. To him, it felt like pieces of the puzzle were coming together, as each speaker chipped away at the enigma of Rh disease.

Adjusting his microphone on the stage, Gorman was now ready to talk about one of the major highlights of the conference: The Sing Sing trials and their successful aftermath. He didn't waste any time making an impression. "Rh immunoglobulin in adequate dosage provides 100 percent protection against sensitization," Gorman said. *One hundred percent.* The only failures that occurred were early on in Liverpool, and had been corrected there. Gorman said that the Columbia trials were expanding and would focus on Rh-negative mothers.

"Currently, Vince Freda has just under five-hundred mothers admitted to our new trial," Gorman said, adding proudly that Presbyterian Hospital had become the world center of Rh research, and that Ortho Pharmaceutical, which was manufacturing the Rh(D) immune globulin, was increasingly optimistic. Thanks to the work of Bill Pollack, Ortho was rolling out Rh trials in forty-three centers in the United States and abroad. He noted that Pollack had at one point even continued the research and Rh production on his own, when funding from Ortho was temporarily halted to be directed elsewhere. But as soon as more data came in, showing the results of the trials, funding was resumed.

The scale of the trials impressed the audience even more. Gorman took a moment to pay tribute to Zipursky, Finn, and others—most notably his colleague and friend Vince Freda—who were working independently but collaboratively on Rh disease. He said there were researchers of note in West Germany who had been inspired by the work of their colleagues Kleihauer and Betke and had begun programs like those at Columbia and Liverpool. The West Germans were the first to demonstrate the effectiveness and safety of intravenous delivery of anti-Rh rather than intramuscular delivery. And in St. Louis, Eugene Hamilton, a doctor inspired by research coming out of Liverpool, had started his own clinical trial, giving anti-Rh injections to mothers following delivery. Only two of his 169 Rh-negative women who delivered an Rh-positive baby were sensitized. Not only that, Hamilton had published results of second pregnancies of treated women. There had been no problems with their subsequent pregnancies.

Gorman delighted the crowd when he shared details of how the protocol of administering the anti-Rh injections within seventy-two hours of delivery came to be the accepted standard for all the clinical trials. "You think it was done through a careful study, research, and analysis, right?" he asked. "Well, not exactly. It was an order from the warden at the Sing Sing prison, where we did our first trials. He set the time at within seventy-two hours to avoid a prison break!" Gorman went on to explain that he and Vince Freda were told in the earliest days of the trial that they would have to vary the days of their returns to Sing Sing to avoid being too predictable. "We could decide which day it would be," Gorman said. "So, the first day we would inject the red cells to boost antibody production. Then we would return within those three days with the anti-Rh.

"We really thought this was a cause for failure," Gorman said. "We didn't want to go more than twenty-four hours before giving the treatment, but we were forced to. And it actually worked fine—and maybe even will give more flexibility to hospitals—to collect the mother's blood at delivery, do blood tests, and give the treatment. We were able to show that it still worked just as well if given within those three days."

Attendees nodded in appreciation, and reporters took notes.

Gorman enjoyed the recognition of their hard work, but he wanted to drive home another important point. He encouraged the scientists and researchers in attendance to always persevere with ideas that others may dismiss or shoot down. His original idea that passive antibodies suppressed active immunity was widely ridiculed and dismissed by the medical establishment. "We were called naïve," Gorman said. "I heard people say, 'That's just Gorman being Gorman.'" Now, unless something went surprisingly wrong, "a discovery of great importance" was close at hand. Taking off his glasses and looking at the crowd, he declared emphatically: "It's working!"

Gorman exited the stage to thunderous applause. *The prison riot. The disdain of the medical establishment. The endless red tape to set up the trials.* It had all been worth it.

The final speaker of the conference was Dr. Gustav Nossal, an immunologist and director of the distinguished Walter and Elisa Hall Institute in Melbourne, run until recently by Sir Macfarlane Burnet. Gorman had hosted Nossal—and Finn, for that matter—at his apartment in Manhattan, where the men would drink martinis and talk into the early morning hours about such things as immunological tolerance and the puzzle of how the body knows not to form antibodies against itself. He and Nossal were both born in 1931 and had both started medical school at sixteen. They had shared early insecurities about whether two blokes from Australia could possibly compete against the best and brightest in America and beyond. Nossal had made one great move after the other, beginning with the mentors he landed in Burnet in Melbourne and Josh Lederberg at Stanford University in California.

Lederberg was thirty-three years old when he won the Nobel Prize in Medicine in 1958. Burnet won the Nobel Prize in 1960.

Nossal, gregarious and self-deprecating, took the stage and began by recapping the key points of the talks by Zipursky, Finn, and Gorman. "They laid out, step by step, their attack on what we know as hemolytic disease of the newborn," or Rh disease. "It is a disease that has taken lives of our most vulnerable, of our unborn children. It is a disease that has robbed families of joy and the generations that would otherwise have followed. But we know that many great things start in tragedy."

Nossal continued, "Scientists need to have a great imagination. They need to dream a little more, a little further, into goals that are meaningful and that exceed their grasp."

Looking at his colleagues and friends and smiling in Gorman's direction, he said, "What we have heard here today is just that—scientists who have great imagination and who have exceeded their grasp."

Then, Nossal said, "You must know, after listening to the esteemed speakers today, that we are in a momentous place and time." He paused for several seconds, feeling a hush fall over the room. He told them: "We do not often have the privilege to be present at the beginning of one of the revolutions in medicine."

The audience soaked up the gravity of the moment. Rh disease was on a path toward eradication. A mystery akin to polio or cholera may have been solved.

Nossal's words were met with a standing ovation.

Reporters rushed out of the building to file stories. Delegates stayed after to talk among themselves. Scientists were eager to report back to their teams. Everyone wanted to be a part of this nascent revolution. One of the next steps would be establishing blood donor programs in communities throughout the world so that women would have access to fractionated blood with the Rh antibodies. There was no time to lose.

Within weeks in New South Wales, the Red Cross blood transfusion committee met and approved funding for the "Rh Project." It would be led by Dr. Baden Cooke, a county blood-bank director with years of experience in general medicine and obstetrics. Cooke had seen the tragic effects of Rh disease in his own practice in Temora and had felt the hopelessness of the Rh mothers he treated who were unable to deliver a live baby. The committee moved fast, determining that conducting its own trials was unnecessary given the strength of the results in Liverpool, Columbia, and elsewhere. The epicenter of the Rh Project would be 1 York Street in Sydney, and John Gorman agreed to serve as consultant and sounding board from New York.

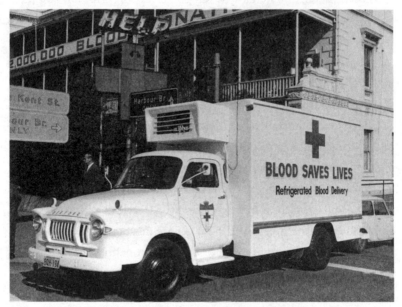

The Red Cross offices at 1 York Street in Sydney quickly became the center of the Rh donor program in Australia.

In one of their first calls, Gorman advised Cooke: "Start the program by getting the women who have Rh disease. Make them your donors. If you don't have enough, start recruiting Rh-negative men."

One of Cooke's first hires was a young woman, Robyn Barlow, who exuded confidence and had arrived for the interview looking impeccable and insisting that her lack of experience in a clinical setting was not going to be an issue. She told Dr. Cooke that she had learned of the job on the train ride back from the airport, where her husband, a helicopter pilot in the Fleet Air Arm, was set to fly with the Americans in the Vietnam War. "I read the ad and thought, 'This is for me,'" Robyn told Cooke. She was hired on the spot.

For Robyn, arriving at 1 York Street was like falling in love all over again. Robyn was enthralled by the building and its history, was charmed by the nurses and donors, and believed in the lifesaving mission at hand. She quickly developed a rapport with Nurse Lizzie and the others and learned as much as she could about blood banking, typing, and Rh disease. She was a quick study.

At night, she read everything she could on Rh disease, underlining and highlighting research material that Dr. Cooke shared. One fact that stuck out for her: "Rh disease was historically one of the major causes of infant mortality and lifelong severe disability in Australia. It had the potential to affect one in every six newborns in Australia—or about 40,000 babies every year."

Robyn was put in charge of recruiting donors, and a letter was sent from the Red Cross to women who had been treated at various hospitals across the country. It began: "Rh babies are newborn infants suffering from anemia and jaundice due to a Rh incompatibility between the mother and the baby. The anemia may be so severe as to cause the death of the baby. Research workers in England, America, Europe and Australia have shown that Rh disease can be prevented by giving all Rh-negative mothers at risk an injection of a special protein obtained from the blood of a person who had been immunized to the Rh factor. The protein cannot be made artificially, and it can only be obtained from persons such as yourself who are known to be immunized against the Rh factor."

It closed with this: "We are writing to ask if you would be prepared to become a special donor so that your blood may be used to help prevent Rh disease."

Robyn asked Nurse Lizzie: "Will the women be hostile? I mean, how would it be to have someone write to you asking for your help when you had just lost a baby?"

Lizzie, who always thought the best of people, said she believed that the women would want to help.

"What about the husbands?" Robyn continued. "Will they be upset with us?"

It wasn't long before she had her answer. The women donors began to arrive at 1 York Street, some looking bedraggled and world-weary, and others with a carefree facade. Most were alone, but a few came with a husband or friend.

Robyn did the intake on every donor to develop a rapport and a bond with each one. No one was paid for blood in Australia. She met a lovely woman who lived south of Sydney who lost her second child to Rh, and then lost her husband to suicide.

One woman who became a donor had lost ten babies to Rh disease. To get to the Sydney blood bank, she had started her day by rowing up a river, walking a mile to the bus, then taking a train to the central station.

These were women, like the "Rh Ladies of Winnipeg," who had watched their babies die or seen them grow up brain damaged or with physical disabilities. Some of the women had been sterilized after repeated stillbirths or neonatal deaths. Robyn made it clear that the experimental treatment in development was too late for them, as it wouldn't work on women already sensitized. But their antibodies could now be used for something great, to try to save lives and help other families have children of their own.

Within a few weeks, Robyn was introduced to Olive Semmler. Olive's Rh-negative blood, heavy with Rh-positive antibodies, had been used for research only, and was classified as unsuitable for transfusions. Olive told Robyn her story of always wanting "a blue-eyed baby," and of the years of losses. Robyn held her hand and asked whether she would turn some of the grief into something good by becoming a donor in the Rh program. Olive's blood was exactly what was now needed to save lives. After talking it over with her daughter, Val, Olive became a part of the regular Rh donor pool. Dr. Cooke had been one of her doctors in Temora.

Robyn told Nurse Lizzie: "You see the tragedy of losing a child. But there are also the dreams that parents have for their baby's life. That loss you don't see."

Dr. Cooke and the team at 1 York Street predicted they would need thirty thousand Rh doses every year in Australia, which meant they would need to recruit up to 1,700 donors.

It quickly became obvious that these already sensitized women could not provide nearly enough of what was needed to protect all the women who would need the treatment. So the appeal was switched to men with Rh-negative blood.

"Look through our files," Dr. Cooke instructed Robyn, "and find any of these Rh-negative donors already in the system."

Robyn soon devised a name for the donors she was seeking. It was MMM—for "Male, Married, and Mortgaged." She wanted men who were stable at work and home and were not likely to up and move.

Gorman had advised them from day one that if they couldn't get enough women donors, they would need to turn to Rh-negative male donors and boost them with Rh-positive blood—just as they had done with the men at Sing Sing. Boosting a donor to produce antibodies could take up to six months.

Sitting at her desk, looking through files, Robyn selected one that appeared thicker than the others. Reading it, she was impressed by the donor's track record; he never missed an appointment. As she read the file, she was struck by something else. His numbers were off the charts. Clutching the file, she hurried off to find Dr. Cooke.

"You must have a look at this one," Robyn said, handing over the file.

Cooke reviewed the records: Rh-negative male with high titers of Rh-positive antibodies. *Very high levels of antibodies.* "Yes, he's a good one alright," Dr. Cooke said.

"And he appears to be just my type," Robyn said with a wink. "Male, mortgaged—I'm guessing—and married!"

A few days later, that "good one" walked through the door of 1 York Street. Robyn made sure she was at the desk to introduce herself.

Seeing a new woman at the desk, James extended his hand: "James Harrison at your service."

Robyn smiled. "Robyn Barlow at your service."

Robyn asked James whether he had a moment to meet with the clinic's director, Dr. Cooke.

"Sure, happy to," James said, suddenly transported to his childhood when he and Ronny and Johnny were summoned to the principal's office. "What's this about? Am I in trouble?"

Robyn said, "I should say not, but I'll let the doctor explain."

The three of them met in Dr. Cooke's office, and Cooke explained to James that "about 17 percent of Australia's population has Rh-negative blood: O–, A–, B–, or AB–. The rest are Rh positive."

James wasn't sure why he was getting an Rh lesson, but he remained polite, as always.

The doctor continued, "Rh-negative women are no different from anyone else, except during pregnancy. If an Rh-negative woman is carrying an Rh-positive child, and that child passes blood cells to the mother in utero, a potentially catastrophic reaction takes place in the mother's body. Her system responds as if her baby's blood cells are a foreign bacteria or virus, and she begins producing antibodies that destroy them."

James nodded, though he had missed about half of what the doctor had said. He was paying more attention to the lovely Robyn, telling himself that even happily married men are allowed to appreciate a good-looking woman.

James perked up a bit when Dr. Cooke started describing the Rh project, and the potential for a breakthrough treatment, something that was the brainchild of several teams, notably an Aussie doctor from Bendigo named John Gorman.

"Oh yeah? That's nice that we've got one of our own," James said.

Robyn explained to James that a new technique called plasmapheresis would separate his plasma from his red blood cells, then his red blood cells would be reinjected back into James to prevent anemia. "The whole process *is* a commitment," she said. "And blood products always carry risks. We would be asking you to come in once a fortnight. You would need to sign papers, and your wife would also need to sign."

Finally, after listening to more scientific talk that went over his head, James cut to the chase: "What are you asking me to do?"

"We want you to be a donor to help women at risk for Rh disease have healthy babies," Dr. Cooke said. "You have the perfect blood for this. *Rare blood.* You already have the antibodies we need to save lives."

James nodded. The idea of helping babies was wonderfully appealing, especially now. He had just learned that he was going to be a father himself. After concerns that his wife, Barb, might not be able to have children, the two had recently conceived. The pregnancy was brandnew, but James could not have been happier.

Robyn thought James was hesitating and said, "You have special blood, James Harrison."

James smiled. In a day, he had gone from having subpar blood—bottled for research only—to having superstar blood that might save lives.

James stood up, shook hands with Robyn and Dr. Cooke, and said, "Sure, I'd like to look after mums and babies. I just need to run it by the wife."

For years, James had pushed aside thoughts that his blood was somehow inferior because it would not be used to save a life, the way those thirteen units had saved his life on the operating table. There were times when coming to the blood bank reminded him of his sickly youth, of the days he was forced to stay inside when his friends were out playing in the street. He saw what was going on around him but felt powerless to act. This never stopped him from giving blood, because it was the right thing to do. But he still wondered whether he was making a difference. Each donation day he told himself, "Living is giving."

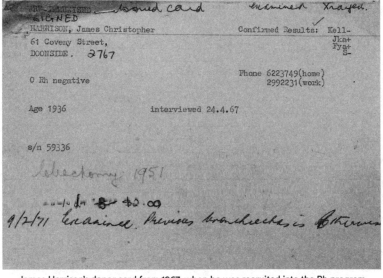

James Harrison's donor card from 1967, when he was recruited into the Rh program in Sydney, notes his "lobectomy 1951."

But now, maybe his father's belief that his blood had been transformed like Peter Parker was true. Perhaps now, at thirty years old, the time had finally come for him to truly return the favor he'd been given as a teenager. Maybe his life was saved so he could do the same for others.

He had little idea just how profound a difference he would make.

CHAPTER THIRTEEN
Lights! Camera! Action!

It was hard for John Gorman not to be nervous as he took his seat behind the desk of the *Today Show* next to Barbara Walters and Hugh Downs. Talking to scientists in Sydney was one thing, but telling the complex story of Rh disease on national television to millions of viewers across America was another.

Walters, in a white suit, glanced down at her notes. Gorman straightened his suit jacket and tie. To his left was Bill Pollack of Ortho. Hugh Downs opened the interview segment by asking what caused Rh disease. The camera moved tighter on Gorman's face, and his name was flashed across the grainy black-and-white screen. Gorman spoke haltingly at first, explaining the blood incompatibility and prevalence of the disease.

Walters asked, "These are the blue babies we hear about?"

"No, that's different," Gorman said. "These Rh babies are actually yellow because of jaundice. The jaundice occurs because of rapid destruction of blood." Pollack then pointed to scientific diagrams showing the destruction that occurs in utero to the baby's red blood cells.

Toward the end of the segment, Walters asked: "Very often with the development of vaccines, there is one hitch, one thing that isn't perfect. Will that be the case here?"

Gorman smiled, looking more confident now, and said, "No, this looks really good. It's been used in male volunteers for three years, and other doctors far and wide have been working on this. It all looks *very good.*"

The guests were thanked, and Downs closed by extolling this "major Rh breakthrough."

Gorman took a deep breath as he left the New York studio. His life had been a whirlwind in the days and weeks following the symposium in Sydney, where he and others had announced major progress in the long fight against Rh disease. His schedule was now filled with interviews, talks, and conferences—a clear sign that the message about Rh had moved from behind closed doors of teaching labs and into the mainstream.

Soon after his national television appearance, his desk became inundated with medical journals, magazines, and articles about the Rh breakthrough. There were also congratulatory cards from colleagues and friends who had seen him on the show or read about him in the latest issue of *Time* magazine. Mostly, though, there were piles of letters. Some of the envelopes were handwritten and smudged, others were meticulously typed on thick stock paper.

Leaning back in his chair, John decided to tackle the letters first. But he wasn't prepared for what he would read.

The first letter began, "Can you help me save my baby?" He scanned the rest and frowned.

The second letter he opened was from a doctor: "I am writing in the hope that you might be able to help me in the management of a Rh patient, now at thirty-eight weeks pregnant." The doctor continued, "The wife and husband are both unusually well informed about Rh incompatibility since she is a trained nurse and he is a hospital pathologist. They both know, too, that the prevention of Rh sensitization is still experimental. But if it were possible to obtain from you a supply of the gamma globulin, enough for her needs, they and I would be most grateful. You could rest assured that your protocol would be followed to the letter."

Gorman opened another envelope: "I am a friend of a former employee of yours, and I believe you may be the only one able to help us . . . My husband and I are expecting our first child and we are Rh incompatible."

And another: "I don't know if there is any hope for me, as I am told that my babies died from Rh."

Some letters included autopsy reports of babies or fetuses, others asked for advice for women anxiously trying to plan for a second pregnancy, and many others inquired about being admitted to a trial. Lives were laid bare.

Gorman organized the letters into categories: doctors, mothers, institutions, and friends of Columbia. Many he would hand over to Vince Freda and the team at the Rh clinic, which was expanding its trials and might be able to enroll a number of the women. Every letter deserved a response.

Sifting through the letters—thin, brittle, fancy—it dawned on him that he had come full circle, returning to the plight of mothers and babies. When he'd arrived in America and started as a pediatrics resident in the Bronx, he was impatient with his patients. The unrelenting questions from mothers felt like challenges. The letters before him were also filled with questions from mothers. The objective, he realized, was the same then as it was now. The women wanted something universal, something at the heart of life: healthy children.

That realization—his growing sense of empathy—was beyond his grasp as a young, shy physician who practically ran away from patients when he first began practicing medicine. But as much as he had changed over the past decade, Gorman in many ways was still the same boy from Bendigo where his own sense of discovery was awakened. His passion had always been building and inventing, moving from idea to invention, chance to significance. Now, as his accomplishments were beginning to draw worldwide attention, it was evident to him that he wasn't in medicine to hold patients' hands, or even save lives—though that would always be a welcome outcome. He was an inventor and entrepreneur who happened to be a doctor. He was interested in the mechanics of medicine. And instead of the dusty shop of his youth, where he fashioned radios from vacuum tubes, Gorman had a university lab and hospital. He had brilliant and dedicated colleagues. But he had always been directed by the same question: *Is there a better way?* Before there was a stethoscope, doctors placed an ear on a patient's chest. Before there were prosthetic limbs, patients had wheelchairs and crutches. Before the invention of the X-ray, there was slicing a person open.

The questions posed by Gorman after reading a few sentences in *General Pathology*—about how the presence of circulating antibody, whether produced actively or received passively, may completely inhibit the immune response—were being answered. Gorman's idea for Rh eradication had moved from a theory that he found beautiful in its simplicity and obvious in its efficacy to an invention moving toward regulation and out of his hands. Plans were underway at Ortho to roll out production and processing. Similar moves were underfoot in various countries involving myriad ministries of health, institutes, and blood transfusion services. In the United States, licensing for the new drug was sought by Ortho from the National Institutes of Health's Division of Biologics Standards, which approved biologic products including gamma globulin. A name had been given to the anti-Rh injection made by Ortho: RhoGAM, a contraction of the Rh antibody and gamma globulin.

Gorman found it interesting that in the field of science, where data-backed evidence ruled, the treatment for Rh still held mystery. No one knew precisely how the passive-antibody-as-medicine suppressed the active immune response. The prevailing "clearance theory" held that when the fetus's red blood cells entered the mother's circulation, the already injected anti-Rh *cleared* the antigens into the spleen and out of circulation, thus preventing an immune response. Another theory held that the existence of artificially created antibodies alerted the immune system that the appropriate response was already in place. One theory was intelligent design, the other more brute force.

Gorman liked the intelligent design explanation from a teleologic viewpoint. He believed that researchers were using an agent designed by nature for this purpose and improved to perfection by evolutionary forces.

Regardless of the mechanism by which the treatment worked, Gorman saw far bigger challenges, notably the recruitment of donors who would need to be artificially stimulated for antibody production. The raw material needed to save lives could not be made in a lab and could only come from 7S gamma globulin containing anti-Rh antibody. The only source was from the plasma of Rh-negative donors sensitized to the Rh factor. He had told blood bankers working on Rh that their first donor group was Rh-negative women who had already been immunized and developed antibodies. Then the blood banks would have to find "very altruistic people who see the need." It was a bit like finding kidney donors. While not as serious, the commitment was long term. And there were the risks. Once the Rh-negative donors were boosted with Rh blood, they were at risk if they needed future surgeries or transfusions. If they were in an accident and given Rh-positive blood, it could be deadly. He knew from his years in blood banking that human errors caused too many transfusion reactions and deaths. And there were risks of getting hepatitis. The hepatitis B virus had been discovered in 1965, and a test for it was in development.

But there was also a unique beauty to this breakthrough. Unlike so many other drugs or medications, this one had not required millions of dollars in research and development.

Drug development was always fraught. The anti-tuberculosis drug Rifampin went through a dozen iterations and excruciating trials with debilitating side effects and unpredictable outcomes over decades, from the study of soil microbes to toxic streptomycin to isoniazid to

Rifampin. Anti-Rh was, as Gorman put it, "a perfectly developed drug" based on Rh, a fully optimized molecule. There was no need for clever chemists to synthesize, fine-tune, and test a novel molecule.

"I hope this is not too good to be true," Gorman had told Vince Freda at the end of the summit in Sydney, when they were all hailed as pioneers. Trials were derailed at every stage. Reaching statistical significance was not easy: The greater the variation in the underlying population, the larger the sampling error. The bigger the sample size, the less likely the results reflected randomness. Only around one in ten drugs made it from clinical trials to federal approval. And getting through phase three of a trial could take years. Gorman compared the expansion of trials to flipping a coin: The more he flipped, the less random the results.

A knock on Gorman's door took him away from reading through the piles of letters. It was Paul Brown, an especially bright young pathology resident who only occasionally made it to classes or labs. In that way, Brown reminded Gorman of himself.

Gorman motioned for him to come in. Brown had graduated from Harvard and then Tufts medical school and had a similar entrepreneurial mind. He had never wanted to attend medical school but did so because his father, a physician on the faculty of both Harvard and Tufts, had wanted his son to become a doctor. "My father made a deal with me that if I went to medical school, he was going to pay for that, but if I went to business school, I was going to pay," Brown told Gorman. "So I went to medical school."

A few months earlier, Brown had gotten a $500 loan from his father-in-law to start a new company. The company would be called Metropolitan Pathology Laboratories (MetPath), with the purpose of overhauling lab work for patients.

Gorman and Brown agreed that the overall quality of lab equipment and processing for patients was terrible and ripe for innovation. Brown opened the lab in his apartment, about ten blocks from the hospital, and Gorman had begun moonlighting as MetPath's director of hematology. When Gorman first went to Brown's apartment in Manhattan's Washington Heights neighborhood, he saw that the bathtub functioned as the staining area for Pap test slides for cervical cancer. Brown's wife was their courier, with their young children in tow. Brown was managing to hire away Columbia Presbyterian staff, including a dozen technicians who did the analysis of pap smears.

"We're going to change the landscape of pathology lab services," Brown told Gorman.

Gorman told his wife, Carol, "This kid has chutzpah." At the beginning of their partnership, Gorman told Brown that he would like a 3 percent stake in the company. Brown said fine, but came back later and told him, "My board won't let you have 3 percent, so you'll have to settle for 1.5 percent." Gorman agreed and now went back and forth to his "lab" to help set up protocols and tests.

A few days later, after getting through most of the letters, Gorman was scheduled to travel to a blood bank conference in Florida. He wanted to show off one of his inventions that had moved from an idea for how to do something better to prototype and now into production. Carol would join him in Florida the following day, so John had to settle for another travel companion. Seated next to him in first class, with its own ticket, was the fifty-pound Electra 500, the new and improved prothrombin time test, which resembled a small suitcase. The Electra had started, of course, as the crude, slow, and inaccurate fish tank contraption at Columbia. After John created a new model using various parts left over from the Manhattan Project, a talented design engineer named Emil Scordato, who had worked on everything from airplanes to elevators and printing presses, was recruited to help. He and Gorman soon cofounded Medical Laboratory Automation (MLA). John was given a 30 percent ownership stake. Gorman and Scordato were convinced that their automated instrument would revolutionize blood-coagulation testing worldwide. Investors began to agree.

The next day, it was Carol's turn to board a plane from JFK to Miami. Though she wasn't officially part of MLA, she was its biggest cheerleader, able to discuss the scientific intricacies of the clotting machine with anyone who crossed her path. Carol had barely settled into her seat when the passenger next to her struck up a conversation, asking whether she was visiting Miami or lived there. Carol told him that she was completing her residency at Columbia to become a doctor and heading to Miami for a medical conference. This information didn't seem to compute with the man, who said he thought she was a model or actress.

Carol, used to being underestimated by men, ignored the comment and told him she was excited about the blood bank conference because they were presenting "a revolutionary new prothrombin machine" that would determine the clotting tendency and timing of blood. She explained the physics behind it, and said it was the first automatic instrument to adopt "photometric principles" to detect the coagulation endpoint.

"It sounds wonderful," said the man, impressed by her scientific knowledge. "I have connections, people who may be interested."

"Well, here's the deal," Carol said. "This machine is a winner. Whoever picks it up will be a winner."

The man didn't need any more convincing.

Carol gave the man her name and John's name and said, "John is well known in the medical field."

The passenger said, "I'm close with Elliott Roosevelt, the son of former president Franklin Roosevelt and first lady Eleanor Roosevelt. Elliott is the mayor of Miami Beach."

Carol nodded but wasn't easily impressed.

When asked how she knew so much about blood, Carol laughed.

"I've had a lot of experience with blood," she said. She told him that when she started as a resident at Columbia, she earned $5 an hour drawing blood. She loved pathology, she said, though she had recently developed a strong interest in specializing in ophthalmology. And she was married to a leading blood researcher.

Wanting to pass the time, Carol decided to tell the man about her unusual honeymoon in New Guinea. "The tribespeople had never seen a white person," she began, "let alone someone with long blonde hair."

"The most unusual thing," she went on, "was that the kids didn't cry when you drew blood. Not one. I've never seen anything like it." She explained that she had directed her interpreter to let the chief know that she would draw blood from him first, to show it was okay and didn't hurt.

"I thought, 'I'll get slugged if I don't get this right,'" she recalled with a laugh. "But I got it right. I put a Band-Aid on—the chief had never seen a Band-Aid. He said something like, 'It's nothing.' He then held his arm over his head like he was giving a victory speech."

Carol's seatmate was captivated. She told him that she and John spent their first night in New Guinea in a motel with twin beds and mosquito netting. John, who had been badly bitten by a nasty bug on a previous visit, wasn't taking any chances this time and made sure the beds were not against any wall. The electricity came and went. "If you put on the light, you could see things crawling up the wall," Carol said matter of factly.

"So the next morning, we go back into the jungle," she continued. "I could not believe my eyes. There in front of me was a beautifully built hut, covered in wildflowers. The chief had ordered the hut built overnight. It was to be my office." That day, one by one, the chief's forty to fifty children were brought in for blood draws, and Carol used her smallest needles. The chief held each child. "They looked up at him with the most beautiful eyes—not one dared to cry," Carol recalled. "I would tell them they were wonderful, and they would smile at me."

She laughed, too, recalling how their driver, who spoke limited English, was the only one she saw wearing actual clothes. He wore the same shorts and a shirt every day. When it was time for John and Carol to leave the island, the driver told Carol that he didn't know what he would do without her and asked whether he could write.

"When I got home, he had written me a letter," Carol said. "He told me how much me missed me and said that if I ever wanted to send him something, he would like just one thing."

"What did he want?" the man asked.

"A pair of long pants!" Carol said, and the two couldn't stop laughing.

As the plane landed in Miami and more contact information was shared, the passenger told Carol that he planned to get in contact right away with the Roosevelts to tell them about the blood-clotting machine. Carol suggested that he reach out to John at the conference.

Within an hour of their flight landing, John, in a closed session meeting, was called out of the room. "The Roosevelts are calling," he was told. "Yes, *those* Roosevelts. They want to meet you." Later that day, John pieced together the mystery of how news of his blood machine had made its way to a Roosevelt. Carol. She was his secret weapon.

When the Gormans returned from Florida, they were happily consumed settling in to their new thirty-ninth-floor flat on East Fifty-Sixth Street, on the southwest corner of the building looking out over Manhattan and the East River. The rent was $600 a month, and John was thrilled with their private terrace. John had been watching the building go up from the window of his previous apartment on Fifty-First and Second Ave. One day after months of following the construction progress, he walked to the building during a lunch break and took the stairs to the fortieth floor. There were still vacancies, and he decided that he and Carol should be on the thirty-ninth floor, in case it flooded. They would soon need the extra space—Carol was pregnant.

The living arrangements were set, which was a relief. The blood-clotting machine was showing huge market potential, which was great. But as the months passed, the anxious waiting period for approval of RhoGAM continued. There were relentless questions from institutions across the globe, and a continued stream of letters and pleas from parents and doctors. Just as Gorman and others were sure they were at the finish line, something pulled them back. The latest stumble came in the form of a failure of an Rh trial in Ireland, requiring Gorman and Freda to fly there to talk to the researchers about what happened. After several days, they discovered that the wrong dosage had been given, and the women involved had become sensitized to Rh. John reminded Vince and others of the rocky path to approval.

Ortho reassured Gorman and Freda that approval of the Rh treatment was imminent. The need was critical—and the market potential was significant. John had looked at the numbers, calculating that if there were five million pregnant women in the United States per year, seven hundred thousand would be Rh negative. Of those, five hundred thousand would have an Rh-positive baby. Half a million babies per year. The number was staggering. The question remained, though, whether to give the RhoGAM only after delivery—the protocol set in place at Sing Sing—or during pregnancy, or both. If RhoGAM were given after delivery, the number of doses needed would be less than five hundred thousand. But if given during pregnancy, when the blood type of the baby was still unknown, an additional seven hundred thousand doses would be required. Johnson & Johnson, the parent company of Ortho, had estimated a $26 million potential annual U.S. market based on the one dose postnatal and noted "the international market could be much larger." The price was set at $64.80 a dose to a hospital lab, with the ultimate cost per dose to patients to be set by individual hospitals.

By using anti-Rh within seventy-two hours of delivery, 90 percent of the cases of Rh disease were successful: the women did not become sensitized. But that left a 10 percent failure rate. Canadian researcher Al Zipursky continued to make the case that anti-Rh needed to be given during pregnancy—ideally at around twenty-eight weeks. Zipursky said that his tests showed there was no harm to the baby or mother, and that 100 percent protection would be achieved by the two doses.

Days stretched into weeks, and weeks into months. The waiting continued. Finally, on a cold winter night in early 1968, John was at home with Carol when he got a call from Bill Pollack at Ortho. John and Carol had both been reading. John listened to Pollack, nodded, said a few words, and hung up.

"Well, any news?" Carol asked.

John sat down next to Carol. "RhoGAM was approved," he said. Carol squeezed his hand. John had told her early in their relationship that it took him all of eight minutes to know that passive immunity would work for Rh. It had then taken eight years for the idea to become reality.

"We did it," he said. "We did it."

CHAPTER FOURTEEN
The First Ladies

"Look at this news!" Marianne Cummins said to her husband, holding up the cover of the Sunday *New York Times*. "An estimated *eighty-seven thousand people* marched against racism and the war in Vietnam in Central Park yesterday."

"This is getting bigger and bigger," said her husband, Dennis J. Cummins Jr., an attorney who represented members of the black community in Paterson, New Jersey, a city adjacent to the couple's hometown of Fair Lawn.

After reading the front-page news, Marianne pulled out the *Times* science section. A story caught her eye—and it wasn't about the war in Vietnam, the assassination three weeks earlier of civil rights leader Martin Luther King Jr., or Hubert Humphrey announcing his candidacy for president.

What grabbed her attention was the headline: "A Vaccine for Rh Disease."

The article began: "This is the story of the long, uphill battle against Rh disease. Last week, after eight years of testing, a vaccine against the disease was approved for marketing in this country."

A New Jersey pharmaceutical laboratory had announced that its vaccine to prevent Rh blood disease had been approved for marketing and would be "generally available on June 1."

It was Sunday, April 28, 1968. Marianne, twenty-nine years old, was Rh negative, and her husband was Rh positive. Marianne was eight months' pregnant—with a due date of May 27. She read the article again. The story explained that the anti-Rh injection had to be given within seventy-two hours of delivery. She looked at the calendar. She would miss it by *one* day.

She read the story aloud to Dennis, who said he'd seen something about it on the *Today Show*. "Ask your doctor about it this week," Dennis said. Until recently, he'd been largely unaware of Rh disease, but he now realized that the condition was a grave threat to their dreams of having a big family.

Their first daughter, Margaret, who was three years old, had been unaffected by Rh—as was the norm with first babies. Their second child, Elizabeth, eighteen months old, was jaundiced at birth, but spent five days in the hospital and fully recovered. The problems were unrelated to Rh. She still had a line in the heel of her foot where her bilirubin was tested. But Marianne knew enough about Rh disease to understand that by a third Rh-incompatible pregnancy, the odds were against them. She would produce the antibodies and probably be unable to have more children.

"The company that makes the medicine, Ortho Diagnostics, is right here in New Jersey," Marianne pointed out. "We cannot miss this by *one day*."

She tore the story out and set it by the door. With two children under the age of three, and her husband running his private law practice out of their converted garage, she had little time to herself. Just getting through the *Times* front page and an inside story was a luxury. As she turned her attention to the kids, she wondered why her doctor had not talked to her about Rh, and whether he knew the release of this lifesaving drug was imminent.

Marianne went to see one of her doctors that week and showed him the story. He said it looked like she would miss it by a day or two. Marianne, incredulous, told her husband later: "He basically said, 'If you can get it, fine. If you can't, fine.'"

Her husband was silent—a sign he was strategizing—and promised to make some inquiries. She too would begin making calls and writing letters.

"Don't wait," she said to her husband. "The baby could come any time."

Marianne and Dennis had met September 2, 1963, at an after-beach party in Bay Head, New Jersey. He told a friend it was love at first sight. They were married ten months later. Marianne, who was the class valedictorian at her college, had just started a job teaching religion and history at a local Catholic high school. Dennis had recently passed the bar. Both were devoted Catholics and socially liberal and had cheered Martin Luther King's "I've Been to the Mountaintop" speech delivered the day before his April 4, 1968, assassination. When the country protested, mourned, and rioted on April 5, Marianne and Dennis joined a massive march in Newark. Marianne, heavily pregnant, pushed her two daughters in the stroller.

Dennis, who believed that his license to practice law should be used for advancing humanity and "honoring everyone's God-given dignity," was known to take on cases that others dismissed as unwinnable. He filed a suit challenging the city of Paterson over its discrimination and mistreatment of black people. Through persistence, he got the U.S. Justice Department involved and won the indictments of thirteen bad cops.

If anyone could get ahold of this Rh medicine, Marianne thought, it was Dennis.

But as the days progressed, and Marianne's five-feet two-inch frame struggled under the weight of the baby, fear usurped optimism. The couple made no progress with their own doctors, and calls to various contacts went nowhere. No one seemed willing to intervene.

Finally, Dennis found a connection, though it felt tenuous. A lawyer he worked with had a live-in girlfriend who worked at Johnson & Johnson, the parent company of Ortho. The girlfriend had attended Dennis and Marianne's wedding, and said she would try to help. Meanwhile, one of Marianne's physicians, Dr. David Landers, also became involved.

Dennis kept up the calls, saying, "Why can't we get this a day or two early?" He had told Marianne early in their courtship about his prolific grandparents. His paternal grandmother had twenty-two pregnancies between 1880 and 1902, with twenty of the babies surviving. His mother was one of fourteen children. Dennis, born during the Great Depression, had only one sister, and told his wife: "We skipped generations. Now it's our turn."

Marianne went into labor the evening of May 26, a day before her due date. Having given birth two times before, she figured she could just go to the hospital in the morning—and not disrupt everyone at night. The next morning, Dennis could see that things were getting serious. Marianne was on the phone with the hospital at seven A.M. and had to stop talking when another wave of contractions hit. As soon as Dennis's mother arrived to watch the girls, Marianne and Dennis got into their Volkswagen bus. The contractions were coming with more urgency, but Marianne still figured they'd be fine. Holy Name Hospital in Teaneck was nine miles away, maybe fifteen minutes by car. And Dennis—who had a habit of walking ahead of Marianne, propelled by his own thoughts—was also known as a speedy driver. They hopped onto 208 South. No problem; traffic was flowing. But as soon as they hit Route 4, they faced a sea of red taillights. It was morning rush hour. Marianne focused on her breathing, summoning every lesson she'd learned in Lamaze class. Dennis focused on the road. He had one thought that he kept to himself: "We're not having the baby in the car."

They made it to the hospital, rushed inside, and Marianne was whisked straight into delivery. Their baby boy came into the world at nine A.M. on May 27. He weighed nearly nine pounds, and looked like "an infant Buddy Hackett," Marianne declared, reminded of the comedian with the chubby cheeks. Immediately after the baby was delivered, his blood was tested, and Marianne's blood was tested again. He was Rh positive. Marianne needed the injection—or this baby would likely be her last. Dennis was on the phone and talking with her doctors. The folks at Johnson & Johnson were now taking his call, and said they were "working on it." They were talking with the United States Public Health Service.

"We have less than seventy-two hours now," Dennis reminded them. After every call that went nowhere, he repeated his personal mantra: "You have to keep fighting to the end." One important factor was working in his favor. He had recently learned that the girlfriend of his lawyer friend was not just some regular employee at Johnson & Johnson. She was the secretary to the president of the giant corporation—hardly a tenuous connection. And she was not letting up, either.

Dennis and Marianne turned to prayer for help, and to give thanks. Marianne was fine, and their new baby was healthy. The RhoGAM was needed to protect the children they still dreamed of having. From the hospital, they worked on the birth announcement. They had named their son Martin—after Martin Luther King Jr. The boy's middle name was John, after the late Pope John XXIII. On the front of the birth announcement would be pictures of Martin Luther King and the pope with the words: "May the ideas of these great men inspire and guide our son, Martin John Cummins."

Monday turned into Tuesday and still no RhoGAM. The Cumminses had twelve hours remaining before it would be too late. Marianne stayed in the hospital with Martin.

On Wednesday, with time running out, Marianne and Dennis learned that Johnson & Johnson had won approval from the U.S. Public Health Service for the early release of the treatment. The couple was overjoyed. A special courier was en route to the hospital. Dr. Landers would do the injection. When the courier arrived and the small vial was brought bedside, Marianne was ready.

As she was rolled onto her side for the injection, Dennis said, "The Lord was with us." The bright and diminutive Marianne Cummins of Fair Lawn, New Jersey, became the first woman in the United States to receive the newly released RhoGAM.

Before the Cummins family could leave the hospital, reporters descended. They wanted to write about the first family to receive this new breakthrough drug making its debut in Teaneck.

News of the first use of the approved treatment traveled fast. In New York, Gorman and Freda were among those who read about the Cumminses' success in getting Johnson & Johnson to release the treatment early. Efforts like the one from Marianne and Dennis Cummins didn't surprise Gorman at all. He knew from the countless letters he had received that determined parents were a force to be reckoned with. Gorman was planning to head to Australia before the end of the year, when a parade would be held in Sydney to spread the word about the new Rh treatment. Nurse Lizzie Thynne was helping the Red Cross

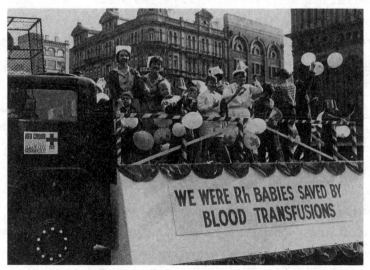

An Rh float was a part of a parade held in the late 1960s to celebrate the breakthrough drug for Rh disease. Nurse Lizzie Thynne (far left, closest to cage) borrowed the rhesus monkey from the zoo.

organize an Rh float, complete with a Rhesus monkey on loan from the Sydney zoo.

After recruiting a limited number of women who had Rh disease into the Rh program in Australia, medical authorities there were focusing their attention on male volunteers boosted with Rh-positive blood. It was clear that the first batch of antibodies from the women would be used up quickly. The Red Cross realized that if the program were to be effective in reducing the number of mothers who had Rh disease, there would also be fewer and fewer women from whom to draw reactive plasma.

So, as Gorman had advised at the international conference in Sydney, sensitization of Rh-negative male donors was underway, with the men injected every five weeks. Australia had proceeded in phases: with the naturally sensitized women, and then with intentionally sensitized Rh-negative males. Given the frequency of injections of Rh-positive blood, there were risks to the male donors. To counter this risk, the donors of the cells to be used were to be sourced in the beginning from just five Sydney donors, who had previously given at least thirty donations that had not caused a transfusion reaction or hepatitis in any recipients. As a further safeguard, before the general program began, the New South Wales Blood Transfusion Committee approved a special clinical trial in which a group of twenty individuals, including some of the directors at 1 York Street in Sydney, were to be given Rh-positive red cell injections themselves to prove the treatment was safe.

The Sydney blood bank then expanded its donor program to include about one hundred forty men—who became the workhorses of the Rh project. Because every vial of blood extracted from the male donors would be used to treat hundreds of women, their blood was closely monitored. These were the men from the MMM group—those who were male, married, and mortgaged.

That strategy was being adopted across the country. In the small town of Cootamundra on the southern slopes of New South Wales in Australia, about two hundred fifty miles from Sydney, a mother named Margaret Thrift had much in common with Marianne Cummins in the United States. Margaret was Rh negative, and her husband, Ken, was Rh positive. Their first pregnancy ended in a miscarriage, but their second pregnancy was successful with the birth of a baby girl in 1966. Now, their second child—their third pregnancy—was on the way, and the Thrifts were told that they would probably need the new treatment made possible by the blood donors in Sydney.

Margaret's doctors had closely followed the story of Rh. Australia's Commonwealth Serum Laboratories had partnered with the Red Cross Blood Service to produce its own anti-Rh called "anti-D"—which stood for the protein on the Rhesus antigen.

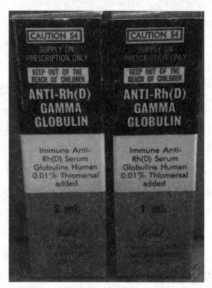

Some of the first vials of anti-Rh, called "anti-D," by Australia's Commonwealth Serum Laboratories in partnership with the Red Cross Blood Service.

For Margaret—like Marianne in New Jersey—having a big family had always been a dream. She worked in a bank, and her husband was a policeman. She had long heard talk of friends or relatives who had "blue babies" or "yellow babies." One of her aunts who lived in Melbourne had a child who had died two months after birth. He was jaundiced and brain damaged.

Margaret was relieved when she gave birth to a healthy baby girl in the spring of 1968. Blood tests showed that the baby was Rh positive. Within seventy-two hours, Margaret received the anti-D injection.

She made her first calls to her parents and her brother to celebrate the newest member of their family. When Christmas rolled around that year, Margaret and Ken packed up their girls and headed home for the holidays. They arrived in Junee with bags and strollers in tow. They were greeted by Margaret's mother, Peggy, and father Reginald—who was dressed as Santa Claus. Standing nearby, beaming and holding his own one-year-old daughter, was her brother, a kind and generous railway administrator named James Harrison. Yes, that James Harrison.

"You look well for someone your age," James said to his sister, ribbing her a bit as was his custom. He put Tracey down so she could run and play and gave Margaret a hug. He asked to hold his new niece, Danielle.

Margaret was sure that it was her big brother's blood that was used to protect her from Rh disease. She believed that the very blood that had saved James decades earlier, when she was all of nine years old, was now protecting their family.

CHAPTER FIFTEEN
"The Switch of a Light"

Behind the wheel of his new twenty-one-foot RV, James Harrison headed out of Sydney in New South Wales toward the Blue Mountains. The pugs, Melinda and Monte, snored in their beds, and his wife, Barb, alternated between watching the road and doing her needlework.

"What are the little ankle biters doing back there?" James asked, looking in the rear-view mirror at his daughter, Tracey, who was now five, and a friend from school who had joined them for the trip.

"Puzzles!" Tracey yelled.

It was a school holiday—meaning that teacher Barb was off work, too—and the Harrisons were out on their first caravan, heading from Sydney to the scenic Blue Mountains and then back to the coast to drive to Melbourne and Victoria in southeastern Australia.

"It's good to leave the city behind," James said. The new RV would be their home away from home, complete with wood paneling, a queen-size bed, bunk beds, and a small kitchen and bathroom. The Harrisons had paid $4,000 for the vehicle, figuring it would be an affordable and enjoyable way to take vacations.

But even on vacation, James could not pass a donor mobile without stopping to give blood. As one of five founding donors of the Australian Rh Project in 1967, James had now been donating for more than five years. He had filled out dozens of forms before being admitted to the program, and he'd even had his life insured by the Red Cross for one million dollars in case anything went awry. When the Red Cross told him of its insurance plans, James said he would talk to his wife. Barb, hearing about it that night, had joked, "Sure! I could use a million dollars, no problem." But after several months of James donating blood, it became clear that he was not being harmed by the Rh-positive injections, so the insurance policy was allowed to expire.

It also become clear to medical staffers that James had remarkable, almost superhuman blood. The blood bank in Sydney meticulously noted his injection dates, titer levels (concentration of antibody), and the amounts of Rh-positive blood injected to boost production of even more antibodies. The average titer level of the Rh-negative male donors boosted with Rh-positive blood was about 400. James's titer levels were ten times that, ranging from 4,096 to 5,120, an amount that doctors found extraordinary—and lifesaving for babies all over Australia.

As James continued cruising his RV through the backcountry, his daughter asked whether they were going to visit Aunt Margaret and Uncle Ken, who lived near the Blue Mountains. Tracey wanted to see her cousins, Kylie and Danielle.

"Not this trip, darlin'," James said. His sister Margaret and her husband, Ken, now had a third child, a boy named Richard, who was going on two years old. The doctors told Margaret that Richard would probably not have been born healthy had it not been for the anti-D injection she'd received after the birth of Danielle. The injection, which she was certain had included James's blood—given he was in every batch made in Australia—had protected Richard from Rh disease.

From the RV window, Barb pointed out the different trees and foliage, the peppermint, silvertop ash, and geebung. As the changing scenery rushed by, Barb served as educational tour guide. Whether cruising over smooth and newly paved highways or bumping along rugged red-dirt roads, James felt grounded. This sense of belonging was new.

For as long as he could remember—he was now thirty-six—James had cycled through different hobbies and interests. When he started stamp collecting, the stamp collecting took over. "Obsessed," Barb would say. "Passionate," James would reply. A few stamps gifted to him in childhood had grown to thousands of stamps in dozens of binders. The arrival of Melinda and Monte had inspired another collection. By last count, James had one hundred-thirty pug items, everything from calendars and pillows to tchotchkes and mugs. After receiving one bromeliad as a gift, his collection grew to several hundred bromeliads that now required a special greenhouse behind their house. "I do go whole hog," he allowed.

But these days, collecting felt a little less urgent. James had arrived at a place where he was secure in his job, family, and community. He was sure he'd found his life's mission. Donating blood cost him nothing but time. He had been told that one whole blood donation could save three lives, but that one donation with the new technique of plasmapheresis could save eighteen lives. To James, that was way more important than any collection.

James stole a glance at Barb and Tracey in the RV. Life felt good. It was similar to how he felt when lifesaving blood transfusions allowed him to be the energetic young man that he had always wanted to be. But this latest feeling of belonging was even more profound. He was now able to share his life with his wife and daughter—and his own life-saving blood with families that he didn't know, and with his own sister.

As the Harrisons neared Springwood, James pointed out the distinctive blue haze surrounding the Blue Mountains. "That's from the oil of the eucalyptus trees," he said. He told Tracey stories of the trains that ran through the mountains, replacing old horse-drawn coaches, and of the first stations located at Emu Plains, Blaxland, Woodford, Lawson, Wentworth Falls, Mount Victoria, and Springwood.

On the road, whenever the Harrisons saw a turnoff that looked interesting, they took it. "We've got a devil-may-care attitude," James said happily. They stopped to get ice cream for Tracey, while Barb and James savored cold glasses of lemon squash—lemonade.

Afterward, it didn't take long to reach the park in the Blue Mountains, where the Harrisons would spend the night. Barb marveled at the beauty of the mountains and the dissected sandstone plateau carved by rivers. "They only look blue until you're in it," she said, "like a trick of the light."

Going to bed late that night, the Harrisons discovered that morning came very early with the maniacal koo-koo-kah-KAH-KAH call of the kookaburras. This was followed by a chorus from the pastel-hued princess parrots and the magpies, which swooped down at the unsuspecting to protect their young. A bit later, there was the screeching and flapping lorikeets—parrots as bright at Tracey's pack of crayons. James swatted at the mosquitos, saying, "Bloody mozzies!"

The vacation was filled with walks, picnics, ice cream cones, and lemon squashes. The Harrisons spotted dozens of kangaroos and wallaby and a few chestnut mice. James alternated between driving along main thoroughfares and country roads with flat grasslands and sheep stations that stretched to the horizon. The family delighted in the unusual names of towns they passed through, from Bete Belong and Wombat Creek to Nowa Nowa and Wy Young. They held a competition to see who could pronounce the name of a tiny rural town called "Bundalaguah."

Days later, as their journey wound down and they headed back into Sydney, melancholy set in. Even the pugs seemed depressed, their normally tightly curled tails uncurling.

James turned to one of his favorite phrases and said, "Don't cry because it's over. Smile because it happened."

After arriving home safely and checking in at work, James announced he was heading to the blood bank at 1 York Street.

Walking in, James was greeted by Robyn Barlow, looking as stylish as ever. "Hello, James—we missed you!"

Nurse Lizzie said hello and began to search for his file. James's records were kept on 5x7 cards. Most of the notes were handwritten, with a few typed. Nurse Lizzie always noted the injection date and antibody levels, and kept track of other antibodies found in the donor's blood, such as the presence of "Anti E-4, Anti E-8, and anti D+C+E."

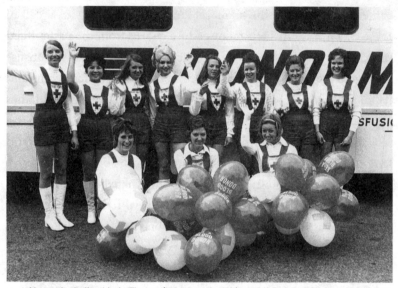

Nurses including Lizzie Thynne (back row, far left), with the Australian Red Cross.

James greeted his fellow donors, and Robyn sat down and listened as James talked about his family's recent road trip.

He's a gold mine, Robyn thought. As a donor, James had never become discouraged when his blood was used only for research. He didn't get upset if he had to wait to be seen by a nurse, or if the nurse didn't hit the vein right away. Some donors up and quit after getting a single bruise. Moreover, very few people had antibodies in such high concentrations. James's body produced a lot of them, and when he donated, his body produced even more. Harvesting his plasma stimulated the production of more plasma, and thus more antibodies. When he'd started donating in the Rh program, he required only a few injections of Rh-positive blood before the anti-Rh antibodies jumped into action.

While James was still talking about his vacation, Robyn excused herself to go and greet one of her regular women donors. She and her husband, a doctor, were Rh incompatible and had four children: The first child was Rh positive and was fine. The second baby was Rh negative and unaffected. The third was Rh positive and required transfusions but survived. The fourth, a boy, survived but was brain damaged.

James and the other donors who remained in the Rh program shared an attitude that what they were doing was simply the right thing to do. A handful of men who had recently become donors did so because of the Vietnam War, which felt like the war that would never end. The donors wanted to do something positive for the country. Robyn had begun to feel a different sort of motivation. She was certain that she was a part of one of the biggest lifesaving discoveries of the twentieth century.

As Robyn walked James back to the blood draw room, she said, "You have become the best donor. You never lose faith in what you're doing."

"I'm just stubborn," James shrugged. "I'm not one to be thrown off course."

Each of Australia's six states had its own blood transfusion center. Robyn and the team at 1 York Street had the largest number of Rh donors of any program in Australia, with about three hundred donors. The Rh programs in Western Australia counted about one hundred donors, and the clinic in Victoria had about two hundred donors.

Robyn had lost her share of donors since the start of the program, and she tried to learn a lesson from each departure. Some donors lost interest, others got sick (unrelated to Rh), a few moved, and others said they feared they could be harmed by the booster shots. Some donors could not be sensitized no matter how much Rh-positive blood they received. To retain donors who had long commutes, Robyn offered to do double donations in one sitting. Though plasmapheresis was time consuming, it would save on visits.

Although Australia, America, Great Britain, and Canada were the first countries to build a donor program and produce their own anti-Rh beginning in the late 1960s, levels of success even in these countries varied. Now in England, only 20 percent of women at risk of Rh disease were getting the shots. In America, it was found that up to three thousand doses annually would be needed per million in population—a number that would require an army of donors donating weekly. Each country was putting together its own estimates of how much of the Rh treatment they would need.

Many governments acknowledged that their Rh programs were years away. Because the anti-Rh treatment was in short supply, the World Health Organization issued a statement recommending that priority be given to mothers delivering their first Rh-incompatible babies.

The problems in getting the treatment out to hospitals and mothers came from stalled bureaucracies, inadequate funding, and challenges in setting up a stable group of donors. Even in the United States, where Ortho had upped its production and lowered the cost of RhoGAM, many women found the cost prohibitive. Appeals for states to step forward with funding for Rh and other public health measures were largely unsuccessful. A bill to lock in federal funding for Rh was vetoed by President Richard Nixon.

Germany and South Africa, while reporting progress in making their own serum, also ran into obstacles. German law, particularly sensitive to medical experiments following the egregious abuses in the Nazi concentration camps, prohibited "the artificial stimulation of humans for antibody production." In Canada, the only donors being used were Alvin "Zip" Zipursky's "Rh Ladies of Winnipeg." They were getting half a liter of plasma a week from each woman, something that was doable through plasmapheresis, the process that kept the plasma but returned the red blood cells to the women. Russia, for its part, had decided that it would only use women who were naturally sensitized and declared it would not take any antibodies from men. In Italy, there was a delay in producing anti-D gamma globulin because of insufficient government funds. Fewer than half of the Italian mothers needing the treatment were getting it.

Women in developing nations went almost entirely untreated. Zipursky and others who investigated the burden of Rh disease in the developing world estimated that there were one hundred thousand newborn deaths a year, with more than twenty-five thousand babies brain damaged. The Australian Red Cross was also looking to see whether it could supply anti-D to women in other countries, including in Southeast Asia.

Despite the obstacles, anti-Rh was making inroads. In the United States, RhoGAM had been given to more than a half-million women since its approval in 1968. In Australia, which continued to try to up its production of anti-D at its own Commonwealth Serum Laboratories, women paid nothing for anti-D. All health care was covered by the government.

Robyn, looking at her watch, returned to the blood draw room to check on James. She wanted to tell him a story a doctor had shared with her about the discovery and use of penicillin. The doctor told her about the day he walked through hospital wards filled with soldiers who were gravely ill. The next day, when the breakthrough antibiotic became available, almost all those men were saved. "Rh is the same," Robyn said. "The switch of a light."

As James and Robyn headed back out to the reception area, James was surprised to see a big group of nurses, doctors, and donors. It was a surprise celebration day. James had reached a milestone. It was June 28, 1973, and he had made his hundredth blood donation to the Rh program. Olive Semmler, standing nearby, had baked a cake for the occasion.

When James walked out of the center that day, he smiled to himself. One hundred was nothing. He was just getting started.

CHAPTER SIXTEEN
A Difficult Dry Spell

"We're going for a ramble," John Gorman announced to his children on a Saturday morning, drawing a mix of excitement and groans, as cartoons weren't over yet. Today's trip would be to the New York Botanical Garden in the Bronx. Almost every weekend, he took the kids on rambles to different parks in different boroughs of the city.

The three children had arrived in three years for John and Carol Gorman: Elizabeth in 1968, John in 1969, and Alexandra in 1970. Elizabeth was the nurturing one, John loved anything to do with science, and Alexandra was an academic star, "competent beyond belief," John would say of his youngest.

The kids brought comfort and joy during an otherwise heartbreaking time. John had recently lost his father, the best teacher he ever had, to pancreatic cancer at age seventy-eight. And in another devastating turn of events, his marriage to Carol, his bright and beautiful fellow adventurer who could charm the tribal chiefs of New Guinea, had crumbled. The relationship that had started with infatuation and mutual respect had ended with yelling and division.

It was 1980, more than a decade since the approval of the landmark Rh treatment that John had helped to engineer. The advance had now saved the lives of countless babies in the United States and throughout the world. But in this stage of his life, at the height of his career, he felt miserable. He was a man of ideas who no longer had his normal clarity, his mojo somehow missing. There were new frontiers to explore, even on the Rh front, and though John was certainly trying to explore them, his ideas were not as sharp. He simply was not himself, not the man who had come up with the audaciously simple concept of fighting Rh with the Rh antibodies themselves.

John hadn't seen the marital split coming. For a man driven to find solutions to seemingly intractable problems, this was a mystery he could not solve, a problem he could not fix. After a decade of marriage, John and Carol were divorced, with John having custody of the kids. He wanted peace, stability, and new routines—and that's what today's outing with his children was all about.

Walking into the botanical garden, John and the kids passed the children's garden and herb garden and stopped briefly to check out the renovations underway at the Enid Haupt Conservatory, long in disrepair. The kids didn't stray far, though, as they could see that Dad was in lesson mode.

His latest teaching moment was what they all called "The Words Project," something inspired by watching Stanley Kubrick's sci-fi film *2001: A Space Odyssey*. John was captivated by Hal 9000, the sentient computer with the soothing voice. He was now writing code and developing software to enable computers to understand English and respond with common sense and understanding.

"Your brains are quite impressive computers," John said as he and the kids walked. "Every concept has a local neuron that is responsive to it, but the way the brain gets to that neuron is very complicated." The kids were doing their best to follow along. They understood that Dad wanted to make computers more human.

John, who was nine—and had the nickname Cito for "little John," as he was the eighth John Gorman in eight generations— thought there was nothing cooler than combining computers and humans. He watched his father start programming, mostly in Fortran but also in Basic. The kids read a *Popular Electronics* story on a new computer kit—the Altair 8800—and always had the newest electronics in their house. They had an IMSAI 8080, an Atari 800, and a CompuPro.

John and the kids headed over to the Peggy Rockefeller Rose Garden. When the hundreds of varieties of roses were in bloom, the fragrance was intoxicating, prompting great sniffing and dramatic oohing and ahhing from one and all. No matter the time of year, there was always something new to see and smell in the garden's two hundred and fifty acres, from the old growth forests to the flowering plants. John loved the bustle of New York, but this wilderness felt a world away from any urban center. Elizabeth pointed to the pale pink blossoming cherry trees and wanted everyone to notice how the same trees were reflected in the pond in the native plant garden. She often told friends that her dad took them on *10-mile walks* every weekend. "And he always talks science," she added.

Cito admired his father's new Adidas sneakers, and thought, *I can't believe my dad has Adidas.*

One of John's recent "assignments" was for the kids to read *An Essay Concerning Human Understanding* by John Locke and try to apply it to thinking about programming a more interactive computer. Cito liked the building blocks of linguistics, telling his dad: "Every idea is a concept." The two talked about how an idea can be pinned down to a uniquely identified thing. "Then you build on that concept," John said. Cito offered: "Take 'cup.' Then 'coffee cup.' Then 'blue coffee cup.' Then 'the blue coffee cup is on the table.'" John nodded and said, "All of the concepts derive from a single one that builds in complexity."

John admired Cito's deep thoughts at such a young age, and wondered whether his son's brain was operating more efficiently than his these days. John had always told his children to look beyond "pedestrian solutions" to find *elegant ideas* that would make the world better. Since the divorce, though, he hadn't had the heart to tell them that he was in a rut. He couldn't tell if they noticed his malaise. After hours of rambling, the Gorman clan was ready for its reward. Here, the kids got ice cream. On the Staten Island Ferry, it had been jelly donuts. Each place had its own treat.

Not long before this latest trip to the park, the kids had gone on their annual six-week getaway to Australia, where they spent cherished time at John's family beach home at Barwon Heads. John's mother, in her mid-seventies, was still practicing medicine. She was planning a trip around the world by herself and was busy with causes focused on the advancement of women. John and the kids visited relatives across Australia—on farms, in coastal towns, and in the outback. John loved America, but he wanted his kids to know their heritage and see the Australia he loved.

As they headed out of the park, John felt this time in nature was restorative. All around was inexorable growth, loss, and rebirth. Nature was about resilience. John surveyed the kids and thought they were doing great—better than he was. He knew this all worked—single dad, three kids—because of their beloved nanny, a Chilean woman named Emily "Emmy" Escanda, who had started with them years earlier. It also helped that the kids had stayed in their home and in the same school. They saw Carol when they wanted, and John was always positive when speaking of Carol. The biggest change for the kids, with Dad in charge, was that they all went out to dinner a lot more.

Finally, arriving home late in the day from the botanical garden, John thought: *Mission accomplished. Kids are exhausted.* After dinner, he got them off to bed and headed into his study. In these moments, the house finally quiet, John often rehashed the unraveling of his marriage. There had been so many good times: dating, wedding, honeymoon, adventures in New Guinea, long talks over shared interests, three wonderful children. Carol was golden like a film star when they met—with a contagious confidence. John was convinced that only Carol could make a prothrombin time test sound irresistible, and land him a meeting with Elliott Roosevelt. The meeting had eventually happened in Roosevelt's grand mayoral office in Miami, where Roosevelt listened, asked questions, and showed great interest, but never invested. Roosevelt was voted out of office shortly after their meeting.

Despite all the happy memories of his marriage, the unpleasant images and fights also played in John's mind. The loss felt tragic.

Before turning off the light, he looked at his calendar, checking the dates for various Rh symposiums. Having his mind off Carol was a good thing. With Emmy in charge, he soon took off for an Ortho-sponsored symposium at the Copley Plaza Hotel in Boston, where the major topic of discussion was the timing of when to give RhoGAM.

After the approval of RhoGAM in 1968, repeated studies showed that giving the injection after delivery was only 90 percent effective, rather than 100 percent effective as seen in the initial controlled trials. Everyone agreed that it was time to revisit the work of the Canadian researchers, including Alvin Zipursky, who had shown that small amounts of the baby's blood crossed the placenta during pregnancy, even without abdominal trauma.

John and Vince Freda had always been spooked by the idea of giving mothers the injection during pregnancy, calling it unethical (and with the real potential for malpractice suits). John and Vince had feared that providing the Rh immune globulin during pregnancy could cause the disease it was meant to prevent. But they, too, had started to rethink their conclusions, given the Canadians' findings of no harm to the fetus.

During all-day meetings in Boston, Canadian researchers Jack Bowman, Bruce Chown, and others revealed that they had gone ahead with injections at twenty-eight weeks into pregnancy, and that their approach was 99 percent effective in preventing Rh disease with no harm to mother or child. They showed that when Rh immune globulin was administered in this way, it did indeed cross the placenta, circulate in the fetal blood, and even coat the red blood cells. But the early treatment, they found, did not lead to jaundice or anemia. The safety was attributed to the low concentration of the anti-Rh given to the mother.

From March 1, 1967, to December 15, 1974, only two of 1,300 Winnipeg women who were given the shots at twenty-eight weeks were sensitized to Rh. The numbers were convincing. By the meeting's end, the all-important American College of Obstetricians and Gynecologists had moved to adopt the twenty-eight-week protocol. Going forward in the United States and wherever RhoGAM was sold, mothers at risk would get one immune globulin injection at twenty-eight weeks, and another within seventy-two hours of delivery.

"There is a 10 percent failure rate" when the shot is not given during pregnancy, John had noted at the meeting. "If we can do better with one in ten, it is absolutely the right thing to do."

When John returned home from the Boston conference, he found the kids buzzing with stories, ideas, drama, and questions. They filled him in on school, friends, studies—and sports. As the months passed, he continued his work as director of the Columbia blood bank. Whenever he started feeling blue because of his divorce, he focused on the good. He had come to the United States with nothing but a suitcase. Now he had made a decent amount of money, had three kids enrolled in the private Dalton School, and he had succeeded in helping to solve the riddle of the global scourge of Rh disease. There were days when he could buoy his spirits, and other days when he felt a heaviness.

In late summer of 1980, John went on a quick trip to England to see his sister Jocelyn. The pair was visiting Oxford when a telegram deemed urgent arrived for John. He took one look at it and was relieved that it had nothing to do with the kids. Yet reading it, he couldn't believe his eyes, and handed it to his sister.

Her eyes grew large. "You won the Lasker Prize!" she exclaimed, knowing that some referred to it as the "American Nobel Prize."

The two sat down for a moment to read the telegram carefully. He had won the Albert Lasker Clinical Medical Research Award, along with Vince Freda, Bill Pollock from Ortho, and the team from Liverpool—Cyril Clarke and Ronnie Finn.

John read what the Lasker folks wrote about his own contribution: "To Dr. John Gorman, for your creative and balanced insight, linking theoretical knowledge of immunology with the therapeutic development of the lifesaving anti-Rh vaccine, this 1980 Albert Lasker Clinical Medical Research Award is given."

He went down the list and read each entry: "To Dr. Pollack, for contributing his immunologic expertise and his knowledge of the fractionation of human serum to the development of anti-Rh vaccine, this 1980 Albert Lasker Clinical Medical Research Award is given."

"To Dr. Freda, for his abiding concern for the mothers and unborn children in his care, which impelled him to seek an answer to hemolytic disease of the newborn, this 1980 Albert Lasker Clinical Medical Research Award is given."

To Ronnie Finn: "For his multifaceted research into the mechanism protecting the unborn child from immunologic attack during pregnancy, for discovering how the weakness of these mechanisms can lead to hemolytic disease of the newborn, and for his vital contributions to the development of the anti-Rh vaccine, this 1980 Albert Lasker Clinical Medical Research Award is given."

And to Professor Sir Cyril Clarke: "For illuminating the genetics of Rh antigen and for initiating and guiding research leading to the potential conquest of hemolytic disease of the newborn, this 1980 Lasker Award is given." The ceremony would be held at the St. Regis Hotel in New York in November.

This time, when John returned to New York, the kids noticed a change: *Dad looks happy.* The *New York Times* announced the news. John was thrilled to be receiving the weighty Lasker winged trophy, which would find a place of prominence on the living room mantel. He was equally impressed by the honorees in other categories. The basic research honorees included Paul Berg, Stanley Cohen, Dale Kaiser, and Herbert Boyer for their contributions to recombinant DNA research. Berg had won the Nobel Prize earlier in the year for his research. John had been following their work in genetic engineering and knew Boyer as a founder of the biotechnology company Genentech.

Back at the blood bank at Columbia, John got the star treatment. His buddy Vince Freda, while happy as well, took days to tell his wife the news of the award, mentioning it only casually one night after dinner. Carol Freda had to laugh. Her husband was motivated not by awards but by the reward of delivering healthy babies.

As the year wound down, with everyone in a more upbeat mood, John and the kids headed to Chappaqua in Westchester County, about an hour's drive from Manhattan, for Christmas Eve dinner. They had been invited to the home of Joe and Barbara Fink. Joe was a friend who worked in the pathology lab at Columbia. Walking in, John surveyed the guests. He knew everyone except one woman—attractive, auburn hair, blue eyes. After drinks and games for the kids, seats were taken. Next to him, he discovered, was the woman he didn't know.

Introductions were made, and John soon learned that Julia Cavalletti, who was from England, lived in a cottage across the street, and was a single mom with a young son named Lorenzo. Julia told John that the Finks were her first friends in America. About halfway through dinner, John realized the Finks were playing matchmaker, and he and Julia were being matched.

John found Julia easy to talk to, and Julia found John wonderfully genuine. When it came time for dessert, Barbara, who was a talented pastry chef herself, made a big deal out of complimenting Julia for making the gorgeous trifle, a traditional English sponge cake. When the trifle was put on the table, Julia noticed John's eyes light up.

Julia laughed. Barbara *was* a clever girl. She clearly had it in mind that Julia would woo this Australian with an English trifle. As John devoured the cake, looking exceedingly pleased with the dessert, Julia winked at Barbara. With the snow gently falling outside and the kids growing tired, John and Julia parted ways. John and family had a long drive back to the city, and Julia had a one-hundred-yard walk to her cottage. Seeing him go, Julia thought, "He's worth a second visit."

Several weeks passed, and Julia didn't hear from John. He had told her at dinner that they were leaving for a holiday, but she feared he might be too cerebral or shy to make a move and ask her out. Julia came from a generation that didn't ask men out but figured she needed to break with tradition. She got up the courage to call, making up a story that she was frequently in New York with her job at *Reader's Digest*, and that maybe they should have a drink.

She rehearsed her lines, placed the call, and reached him on the first try. She delivered her lines and waited. There was a long pause on John's end.

Finally, after what felt like an eternity, John said, "Oh, that would be very nice." Then after a longer pause, he offered, "Maybe we could have dinner."

"Dinner it is," Julia said, relieved.

So, on a Friday evening in early January 1981, John and Julia met for dinner in Manhattan. They talked about families, kids, and lives back home in Australia and England. "I had this beautiful childhood house," she told him. "My parents lived in an old watermill house. I have wonderful memories of climbing the watermill."

It was late when the two said good night, with John returning to his flat and Julia starting the drive back to Westchester County. *He's a nice guy*, she thought to herself as she got onto FDR Drive along the East River. The evening had gone beautifully, and the conversation flowed. But just as she picked up speed, shifting into higher gear, the clutch cable on her Fiat snapped. She tried to stay calm and maneuver over to the shoulder. There were no pay phones in sight, but there was a hospital across the way. She realized she would need to take her life into her hands and sprint across busy FDR Drive. She was breathless when she made it into the hospital waiting room. She fished John's number out of her purse, and dialed him, aware of how late it was.

"I'll come to get you," John said, "and we'll have to get your car towed."

About two hours later, the car was finally taken to the repair shop, but the stranded Julia had no way back to Chappaqua. John said she could spend the night at his house. "This is turning into quite the memorable first date," Julia said. John smiled and said, "Yes, it is." Once home, he got Julia blankets and suggested that she sleep in one of the beds not occupied by the kids. The next morning, Julia emerged with a blanket wrapped around her, in search of the bathroom. She bumped into Elizabeth, who was playing on the Atari.

"Oh, hi," Elizabeth said nonchalantly, unfazed by the sight of Julia. Later that morning, after the kids had been fed and the nanny had arrived, John took Julia to the railway station to catch the train to Chappaqua. As she waved goodbye to John, she was sure she saw something changed in his expression. *I think he may be smitten*, Julia said to herself happily.

She was right. Within nine months, John and Julia were married. When it was time for the wedding rehearsal, Julia declared: "We're all a part of this marriage. We're all walking down the aisle together." Three Gorman children, one Lorenzo, and two adults. After the wedding, Julia and Lorenzo moved in with John, Elizabeth, Cito, and Alexandra.

Julia had known nothing about Rh before meeting John. She'd never heard of it, but she had come to understand the breakthrough by

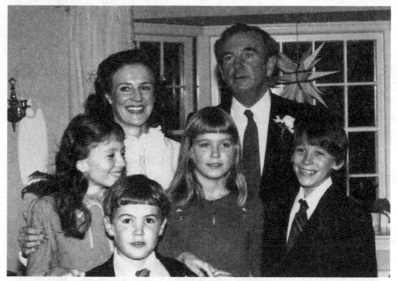

John Gorman and his wife, Julia Gorman, shortly after their wedding, with (left to right) John's children, Alexandra, John (Cito), and Elizabeth, and Julia's son, Lorenzo Cavalletti.

thinking of it this way: John had figured out a way to trick the mother's body into thinking it had already made the antibodies, so she didn't have to make them herself. She found John brilliant and loved hearing about his different projects.

The two were soon invited to an Rh conference in Edinburgh, where one of the main agenda items was whether England would adopt the twenty-eight-week protocol, as the United States had recently done. A grand evening event was held in a beautiful hall in the Edinburgh Castle, with the British scientists indulging in lengthy self-congratulatory speeches, toasts, and roasts. John listened with interest as the discussion focused on costs and benefits of moving to a twenty-eight-week protocol.

To John's shock, as discussions waged on, the scientists were concluding that it was too expensive to give the treatment at twenty-eight weeks into a pregnancy. One scientist summed it up by saying: "There aren't enough failures. It's not worth the money."

"This is just wrong," John said to Julia as they left the hall that night. Julia was fuming over something else. The evening was filled with effusive accolades and encomiums for the team from Liverpool. Everyone knew that John Gorman was in attendance, yet his name didn't come up once all night. "This was a real snub," Julia said to him. "This wasn't a race. This was two groups on different sides of the world working on the same problem."

"There is no excuse for you not to be recognized," she said. John didn't take the English slight personally, but he had to admit that he liked the feeling of Julia being protective of him.

The next morning, John got wind of a surprise decision. After the scientists had turned down approval of the twenty-eight-week protocol, several politicians, BBC journalists, and members of Parliament had called an emergency meeting. The bottom line was: "If you are told you can cut the other 10 percent—potentially save more babies—then we have to do it."

John was surprised and delighted, telling Julia: "The non-medical people are the ones who said we are going to do that. The political decision was the right one, and the science decision was the wrong one!" Julia listened but was still miffed that John was entirely omitted from the program.

Back home, Julia's British influence on the family began to take hold. Elizabeth started calling their family "very beverage-centric." When John and Julia woke each morning, Julia brought tea. Tea was often served again at four P.M. John would then roll into his favorite beverage—a dry martini. Then it was dinnertime.

There were days when John would disappear into this study consumed with his latest projects, only to emerge at two P.M. Julia would say, "You better go to work, otherwise you won't have time to get there and back for tea!"

One of the things that Julia loved most about living with John was having tea in bed. For John's part, he loved Julia because she was both reliable and an inspiration, a woman who had finally put an end to his difficult dry spell.

Almost every morning now, he woke up and said to her, "I've just had a wonderful idea."

CHAPTER SEVENTEEN
A Showstopping Performance

For attendees of the medical conference in Hobart, Tasmania, it was enough just to be hearing from the man who had been instrumental in developing a treatment for Rh disease. But as he approached the stage of the ballroom in the Wrest Point Hotel, John Gorman had a surprise in store for everyone: a special guest who wasn't listed on any program.

Today's speaking engagement was the main event of a trip to Tasmania for John and his new wife, Julia, who had spent several wonderful days of sightseeing mixed in with the medical meetings. John and Julia had walked above the forest canopy on swinging bridges, gone to wineries, hiked to see the roiling junction of the Huon and Picton Rivers, played golf, and taken in the views of the Tasmanian wilderness.

In the ballroom, medical authorities from Singapore, Australia, New Zealand, and across South Asia had no idea about the force of nature awaiting them, nor did the force of nature herself have any idea that she was going to be part of the program. But as John arrived at the dais, it was first things first: the story of immunology and the conquest of Rh disease.

"Rh disease of the newborn is quite rare today," Gorman began, "but before RhoGAM, it was a disease that caused fetal mortality and morbidity in the practice of every obstetrician."

Using Kodachrome slides, he shared the story, from his idea for a treatment to the trials at the notorious Sing Sing prison to the licensing of RhoGAM in 1968.

"In 1960, Vince Freda and I proposed using passive anti-Rh antibody to prevent sensitizations in Rh-negative mothers," he said. "At the same time and quite independently in Liverpool, Ronnie Finn and Cyril Clarke made an almost identical proposal and began a project of similar design. The proposal was to give the Rh-negative mother passive antibody at the time of delivery and thus render her unresponsive to the antigenic stimulus she might receive from Rh-positive fetal red cells entering her circulation."

Gorman explained in detail how the incidence of Rh disease could not immediately drop to zero because there were reproductive age women sensitized before the treatment was introduced— five hundred thousand in the U.S. alone—and these women were continuing to bear Rh-affected babies.

What remained elusive and frustrating, Gorman noted, was the need for "more complete public health planning so that protective coverage on a worldwide scale is available to every woman who needs it from her first birth to the end of her reproductive years."

Gorman, Freda, and others involved in the Rh battle had been dismayed to learn that use of anti-Rh in developing countries was almost nonexistent. "If Rh hemolytic disease of the newborn is to be eradicated, new sensitizations must be prevented," he told the crowd. "The price is constant vigilance, with more efficient laboratory monitoring and management procedures installed to ensure 100 percent utilization of Rh immunoglobulin. Every Rh-negative woman at risk of exposure to Rh positive blood must be covered with an adequate dose."

"We can eliminate Rh disease across the globe," he declared. "In the United States, RhoGAM is estimated to produce savings in human and financial costs exceeding $750 million annually." Then he said, "The Rh treatment has a track record of being one of the most effective and safest products in the history of vaccines."

Gorman put away his presentation notes, tucked his glasses into his suit pocket, and looked out at the audience. He searched the room and nodded when he finally found the special guest he was looking for—way in the back.

"Now I want to share with you," he began, "a personal story, the story of the first pregnant woman anywhere in the world to receive RhoGAM—*four years* before it was approved." Attendees perked up. "I want you to meet my sister-in-law, Kath Gorman. Kath, would you stand up?"

A spotlight searched the back of the room. Kath, taken by surprise, reluctantly stood up and forced a smile while thinking, *John, I'm going to kick you for this!* She was there with her husband, Frank, John's brother.

"Go ahead and ask her your questions," John directed the audience. "She had the injection in 1964 and is here to tell the story."

Hands started popping up. Kath wanted to kill John.

First question: "Why did you agree to do it when there was a lot of risk?"

"I didn't have a bloody clue—I just went ahead with it," Kath said, prompting great laughter.

When the laughter died down, she explained that she'd been in premature labor the day she and Frank went to Heathrow Airport in London to pick up the container, "shipped like contraband" from New York by John and Vince Freda.

She said, "But you asked why I agreed to it even though there was a lot of risk. Well, we were certain it wouldn't harm the baby, as the baby would already be out, and we were pretty certain it wouldn't harm me. But I was the guinea pig for sure."

She continued, "We did it because we had faith in John. We all had faith in John." John, still at the front of the room, was touched by the words. "We knew we wanted more kids, and this sounded like the only possible way for us." Then, looking at her husband and nodding toward John at the front of the ballroom, she added, "Besides, when the Gorman men take over, that's it.

There was more laughter. John was quite aware that Kath had always been a clever girl who was quick with a joke, but he couldn't help but admire how she had the audience eating out of her hand.

"In the end, the doctors at the hospital—not knowing what to do really—called the guys from Liverpool," Kath recalled. "They could have stopped it, but they eventually said, 'Go ahead.' They weren't going to do anything to stop it."

"What were you thinking at this point?"

"I was thinking maybe we'll get another baby out of this," Kath said.

As John listened, he was struck for the first time by the daring of his transcontinental shipping of human serum to be given to a pregnant woman—to his brother's wife—in another country. He thought to himself, "We were wild-eyed optimists."

Another hand shot up. "How many children do you have?"

At this, Kath smiled and said, "How much time do we have?"

"There is Kieron—Kieron Francis Gorman—the first baby, who was born on January 31, 1964. He was Rh positive, so that's when I got the American shot in the English hospital." She added, "Kieron was fully toilet trained by twelve months, and when he first talked, he talked in sentences." There were appreciative nods, especially from the mothers in the room. "He was a very intelligent child."

"Then we adopted a baby boy named Ian, not knowing if we were going to be able to have any more," she said, now speaking into a microphone that someone had rushed to the back of the room.

"But then came Angus in 1965," she said of their second baby and third child. "We called him Angus because he screamed like a bull."

More laughter.

"Then we had the third baby in 1966. A girl. She was a big baby. We thought it was going to be another boy and had picked out the name

Karl. Frank was out of the country, and he rang me up at the hospital, and I told him we had a girl. An hour later, Frank called again and said, 'We have a girl, do we? What are we calling her?'"

"I said, 'The nurse suggested Kirsten or Ingrid, and I like Kirsten,'" she said. "And so now we had four children under the age of three." Both Angus and Kirsten were Rh positive, requiring Kath to get the treatment after delivery, as she'd done with Kieron.

As the crowd started clapping again in appreciation, Kath held up her hand.

"The next baby was Friedel," she said, to wild applause. "Friedel was a big baby. She had jaundice at birth. Her skin was bright yellow. I remember they put her in a big crib and had her dressed in a pink bonnet and booties and a pink onesie, and she looked terrible." The doctors said the jaundice was unrelated to the Rh factor.

"She needed a blood exchange, and then once she had that and started feeding, she was fine," Kath said. "All my babies were good feeders."

John watched with amusement. Kath had stolen the show.

More hands shot up, but Kath said she wasn't done with her last answer.

"Next came Giles," she began, prompting more applause. "He was ten pounds, eleven ounces, gorgeous. Our only blonde." He, too, was Rh positive.

Kath said, "Giles had these beautiful golden curls. One night my four-year-old decided to cut off his curls in the night. I went in to check on him in the night and felt this hair in the crib. I put the light on, and there were his curls!" Kath shook her head. "I don't know how she did it through the crib rails. It's a miracle she didn't cut him. I asked her the next day, 'Did you cut Giles's hair?' She said, 'Yes, mum.' 'Why did you do it?' 'I felt like it,' she said."

"Then came Master Jacob," she continued. "He weighed eleven pounds, five ounces. Before he was born, Kirsten and Kieron fought over whose baby it was. They would feel him kick in my stomach and claim him as their own. When he was born, he was doted over like you can't imagine. They would take turns fighting for who got to bathe him and watch after him. He's a good, sensible boy."

She added, "I was pregnant with Jacob when the cyclone hit Darwin." There were nods of recognition. Cyclone Tracy had hit Darwin early on Christmas Day 1974, killing seventy-one people, injuring hundreds, and devastating 80 percent of the city. It was one of the most destructive cyclones to hit Australia. "Our house was on stilts. We were all in the first level, which held. The level above us was wiped away. We emerged to see our mattresses in trees, clothes everywhere. Every house was destroyed. But we were all fine. The kids were all fine. That was all that mattered." Kath got quieter, telling the crowd that she'd had the injection with every baby. "I had a 50 percent chance of having an Rh-negative baby, where I wouldn't have a problem," she said. "But we kept producing the Rh-positive ones. I was able to have six healthy babies because of these injections."

She added, "Kieron, our first, is now twenty. He's going to be a doctor—so he can save lives."

Looking toward John at the front of the room, she said, "We got healthy babies. We got the big family we wanted, the Christmases with kids all playing on the floor, with busy happy times. Can't ask for anything more now, can we?"

Table by table, attendees rose to their feet and applauded. Some people were crying—including John.

John could talk all day about Rh disease, immunosuppression, passive antibodies, cell clearance, clinical trials, sensitization, titers, and more. But all of it came down to what Kath had so beautifully shared. In the end, it was about healthy kids playing on the floor at Christmastime.

CHAPTER EIGHTEEN
One of Their Own

At the Red Cross center in Sydney, Robyn Barlow and Nurse Lizzie navigated through a throng of protesters, quickly making their way inside the building for an emergency meeting. It was a chaotic and scary period. Hysteria had taken hold everywhere, from big cities to small towns, from Australia to America—and blood banks were not immune from it.

The crisis had its origins in 1981, when a rare lung infection was found in five previously healthy gay men in Los Angeles. Farther north, in San Francisco, yet more patients were reporting rare skin lesions called Kaposi's sarcoma. Those who got sick, mainly gay men or intravenous drug users, were wasting away and dying terrible deaths.

The incidences of the mysterious ailment quickly multiplied, and soon, the malady had a name: AIDS, for acquired immunodeficiency syndrome. During the next several years—as it was discovered AIDS was caused by a virus, HIV—panic spread to communities, schools, offices, and hospitals across the world. Hospital workers donned infectious disease suits. Patients were isolated, with Do Not Enter signs placed on their doors. Some hospital beds went unchanged, and food trays piled up as nurses and staff were afraid to get sick themselves. Family members shunned infected family members, customers at bars were afraid to drink out of a glass used by a gay man, and rumors circulated that the virus was spread through everything from teardrops to mosquitoes.

In Australia, a national television ad featuring the Grim Reaper terrified citizens of all ages. The ad featured the black-cloaked personification of death in tattered clothes and decaying flesh, and an ominous voice: "First only gays and IV drug users were being killed by AIDS. But now we know every one of us could be devastated by it. The fact is over fifty thousand men, women, and children now carry the AIDS virus. In three years, nearly two thousand of us will be dead. If not stopped, it could kill more Australians than World War II." The ad showed men, women, and children being struck dead with bowling balls as they were lined up as human pins.

It had become clear that AIDS wasn't a disease limited to homosexuals and drug users. Transplant patients and hemophiliacs were becoming infected with HIV through contaminated blood. The reality hit: HIV could be contracted through ordinary blood transfusions, putting everyone at risk.

The Centers for Disease Control and Prevention in the U.S. convened a special session to discuss what measures should be taken to protect the safety of the nation's blood supply. But leaders of the blood-banking industry around the world had been reluctant to accept that AIDS was spread through blood, and slow to adopt precautionary measures. At the New York blood center, a director said: "We must be careful not to overreact. The evidence is tenuous." Likewise, a professor with Australia's national blood transfusion centers weighed in, saying that there was "no risk" of contracting AIDS from blood, because Australia relied on voluntary donations and never paid for any donated blood products.

Yet in a decision that mirrored a policy adopted in the U.S., Sydney blood transfusion director Gordon Archer took a cautious approach. He called for homosexual blood donors to voluntarily stop donating, a move that prompted accusations of discrimination and bigotry. Dr. Archer said in a television interview that it was "a virtual certainty that AIDS was in the blood supply." In response, activists picketed the Sydney center and handed out leaflets that read, "Ban the Bigots not the Blood." The demonstrations pained Robyn and Nurse Lizzie, who sympathized with the protesters but thought that Dr. Archer was working in the best interests to protect the country's blood supply.

Arriving inside the blood center, away from the protesters, Robyn, Lizzie, and the team in Sydney held their own emergency meeting to go over new procedures around interviewing donors—including questions around sexual identity and sexual practices—and the use of protective gloves for all blood injections and blood draws. The staff reviewed the new heat treatment methods for ensuring that the blood products used for hemophiliacs were safe. Doctors from Sydney had discovered these methods from a young virologist at UC San Francisco, Dr. Jay Levy, who had been one of the first to isolate the AIDS virus. Levy also had developed an antibody test to detect infection by HIV and was among the first to use heat treatment at 140 degrees Fahrenheit (60°C) for seventy-two hours to inactivate the virus in collected and stored blood.

For blood banks like the one in Sydney, the challenge was not only explaining to blood recipients that steps had been taken to make the blood supply more secure; it was also about reassuring the donors themselves that they would be at minimal risk. This was particularly important for keeping intact the Sydney blood bank's Rh program. Robyn emphasized to the donors in the Rh program that the booster shots with Rh-positive blood used to stimulate antibody production were safe. She reminded anyone who asked that the antibodies used for the Rh injections went through blood fractionation, separating it into component parts, and largely came from the same pool of donors she'd had since 1967. She took pride in her MMM group of male, mortgaged, and married. And she touted the ongoing dedication of her women donors who continued to give, who made their way to Sydney through bad weather, long journeys, and now picketers, scare tactics, and new and invasive forms to fill out.

Eventually, the protests outside the clinic became less frequent, before dissipating altogether. The frightening TV ads went off the air, and calm seemed to be restored. But then more bad news would hit. The latest devastating report, confirmed by the government, was that three infants had died in Melbourne after receiving contaminated blood from an HIV-positive donor.

But donors in the Rh program, ever dutiful to the mission of saving babies, kept giving blood. "I've only lost two donors," Robyn noted, keeping her fingers crossed that no more would depart. The ones who left told her they were no longer confident in the country's blood supply.

James Harrison never wavered during the crisis, arriving at the blood bank like clockwork. "No stopping me," he told Robyn. "I trust you with my life." His certitude and dedication made Robyn tear up.

"Even with all of this chaos, we need to plan our twentieth-anniversary event," Robyn announced one day in 1987. "We need it now more than ever, to celebrate the donors who are sticking with us. I've got fifty of our original donors still with us." She singled out women for special recognition, reminding everyone of how they continued to give after years of losses, including Mrs. Grant, two live births from eight pregnancies; Mrs. Cuddihy, one live birth from four pregnancies; and Olive Semmler, one live birth from seven pregnancies.

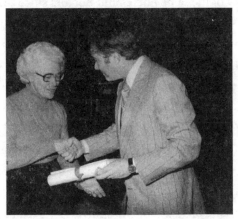

Olive Semmler lost multiple babies to Rh disease before learning that her antibodies could be harvested to prevent other women from suffering the same losses.

So in June 1987, Robyn and the blood transfusion center team held an evening event to celebrate the twentieth anniversary of the Rh project in Australia. Everyone welcomed a night of good news. Dr. John Smith, one of the directors said, "These donors volunteered out of altruism." Each donor received a Red Cross Service Award.

Dr. Gordon Archer told the group, "We are proud of our Rh Project and we are very proud of you." He went on, "The donors here and at the center in Perth have provided nearly all of the anti-D needed to make the project completely effective in Australia. No woman who has needed anti-D in this country has had to go without it since 1969, when Australia became the first country in the world to make it available without restriction, and of course, without cost to the patients."

Robyn had developed close relationships with all the donors, learning about their jobs, families, hobbies, vacations, and dramas. She understood that part of the beauty of the Rh program was that the donors knew that their blood was going into a pool to save the lives of babies and give hope to families from all walks of life. They had a shared sense of purpose. "That's why our product is safe," she said. "We have the same donors in every pool—every batch—ever made." They even had many of the same nurses and doctors since the inception of the program.

They also celebrated—with only a hint of sadness—their move from the building they loved at 1 York Street to a new location on Clarence Street. They now had a bigger ward with five beds, an office, a storeroom, and a small laboratory to house refrigerated products. "No more feet sticking out the window," James had said. "I'll miss that." The blood transfusion service took over the first three floors of the new site. Everyone liked to say, "You can always find Robyn as there's a path worn to her door."

Toward the end of the twentieth-anniversary event, a special honor was reserved for one donor.

"James Harrison, come on up," announced Dr. Archer. James was being recognized for his four hundredth donation. When asked to give a speech, he demurred in his usual way, saying, "I just keep showing up. That's my one and only superpower."

After the event, James and Robyn got a chance to catch up.

"You look especially happy," Robyn said to James.

"Yep—Tracey is off and married," James said of his daughter. "Good husband. I know the parents. They were married at the Blacktown Uniting Church. He works for the department of agriculture, and Tracey is at the railway." He showed Robyn a photo of himself and Barb with Tracey on her wedding day. James wore a dark blue suit with a gray tie, Barb wore a pale blue dress and hat, and Tracey looked gorgeous in a scoop neck wedding gown, a strand of pearls, and a veil.

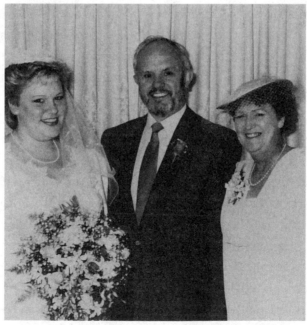

James and Barb Harrison with their daughter, Tracey, on her wedding day.

"That bouquet is beautiful," Robyn said, studying the flowers that Tracey held, with fuchsia, pale pink, and white roses. James had a pink rose in his lapel. "I look pretty handsome, now don't I?" James asked with a wink.

Robyn wanted to know all the details. "How did they meet?"

"Andrew was one of Barb's students at the high school," James said. "I guess a few years back, he sent Tracey a flower on Valentine's Day, but didn't include a card. When Tracey recently had that surprise twenty-fifth wedding anniversary party for us—you were there—he was there, too. She straightaway asked him about the flower, and that was that."

James reflected on how fast Tracey's childhood had gone, from their early caravans around Australia with the pugs to her high school years and now marriage. "The blink of an eye," he said, from taking her to buy her first softball bat, to her dance lessons and recitals, to her playing the organ. One day he was holding her small hand in his as they crossed the street. The next he was walking her down the aisle.

He and Barb had been unable to have more children. They had explored the options of adoption and foster parenting, but never found the right fit.

"I feel like I watched her grow up," Robyn said.

"She's a good girl," James said wistfully.

Robyn clasped James's hands.

Tracey had always loved visiting the blood bank with her dad. She found Robyn "movie star glamorous" and never tired of hearing Nurse Lizzie tell her latest stories about her birds and chickens. Tracey asked Nurse Lizzie every visit to tell her how she could possibly iron with a chicken up on the ironing board. Tracey had also been fascinated by the center's plasmapheresis machine, which she called "the washing machine," as it took her dad's blood, collected the plasma, and returned the blood cells. She could see the way the nurses fussed over her dad.

But her favorite thing was their family routine after the blood bank. She and her father always stopped for milkshakes.

For James, the years continued to fly by. Barb retired from her job at the high school in 1992, after twenty-five years of teaching. James retired from the railway at age fifty-five. It gave him more time with Barb, time to organize his wine collection, to care for his bromeliads, and to continue donating blood. He and Barb were building a house in Umina Beach, about an hour north of Sydney. Tracey and Andrew, who were living in the lower unit of the Doonside house, would eventually live there on their own.

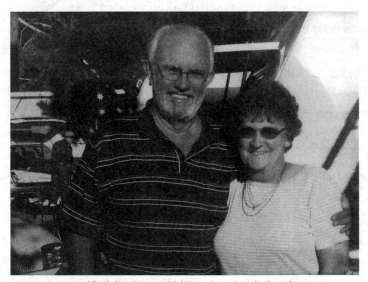

James and Barb Harrison couldn't have been happier in retirement, and they loved caravanning around Australia in their new RV.

Then, in short order, came more good news: James and Barb were going to be grandparents. Tracey and Andrew were expecting a boy.

"Have your blood type checked," James told Tracey. As it turned out, to everyone's surprise, she was Rh-negative, and Andrew was Rh-positive. They could have the same problem that James had dedicated himself to fighting. Tracey would need anti-D.

"See, your good old dad does know best," James said. As soon as baby Jarrod was born, Tracey got a shot of anti-D. The Rh protocol in Australia at the time called for only one injection after delivery and had not yet uniformly adopted a second injection at twenty-eight weeks. Tracey was told that she would probably need the Rh treatment with each pregnancy.

And soon enough, another baby was on the way. Robyn, hearing the news, had called James to tell him: "We may have a problem."

"As you know, because of the AIDS scare, we had to stop boosting our donors," Robyn said. "We couldn't hyperimmunize them the way we always did—and the situation has only gotten worse. We need to do multiple tests on the collected red cells, and then freeze them for a period. Each batch must be tested three to four times over the course of a year. And the officials keep throwing new tests at us all the time. As you know, you must keep boosting or you can't keep the antibodies strong enough. So, our supply of anti-D is about down to zero."

In the eighties and nineties, the AIDS toll had continued to climb. In the U.S., Ryan White, a thirteen-year-old hemophiliac who had contracted AIDS from a blood transfusion and was barred from school in Indiana, had died. Other notable deaths included Rock Hudson, Liberace, Robert Mapplethorpe, Freddie Mercury, Arthur Ashe, Rudolf Nureyev, Keith Haring, Halston, Elizabeth Glaser, and Randy Shilts. Earvin "Magic" Johnson announced he had HIV in 1991. There were occasional positive developments, including approval of the first anti-HIV drug, AZT. Yet at $10,000 for a one-year supply, AZT was the most expensive drug in history. John Gorman had left Columbia in New York to work as head of the blood bank at New York University. It was the NYU blood bank—before Gorman's arrival—that had unknowingly provided HIV-infected blood used in Arthur Ashe's open-heart surgery.

"You know that by 1990, nearly twice as many Americans had died of AIDS as died in the Vietnam War," Robyn said. She and her colleagues at the blood bank had all followed news of the massive march on Washington, D.C., for gay rights. A giant AIDS quilt—with panels celebrating the lives of people that the disease had claimed—was displayed on the National Mall. And now, by 1994, AIDS deaths had reached an all-time high. There had been 441,528 cases of AIDS reported, and 270,870 deaths.

Each country was reeling from the fallout of contaminated blood that had claimed lives, devastated families, and prompted crippling litigation. Although AIDS was first reported in Canada in 1982, it took three years for the Canadian Red Cross Society to start screening for HIV. Australia, England, and other countries were dealing with thousands of people who were infected before safeguards were put in place. Hemophiliacs, who needed regular blood treatments, had filed lawsuits after being exposed to blood plasma contaminated with HIV, hepatitis C, and other viruses. In many cases, blood products from the United States were to blame, as blood had been collected for years from prisoners, drug addicts, and other marginalized groups who were paid to donate. Many blood bank directors were finally forced to acknowledge they had failed to safeguard the blood supply and protect the most vulnerable patients.

"What does this mean for Tracey?" James asked.

"It means we have very little anti-D—at least produced by our group, by Australians—left in all of Australia," Robyn said. "Without the boosting, we don't have strong enough antibodies. If the titer of the antibody is too low, it won't protect the mother."

Robyn promised James that she would do research on the availability of anti-D. She soon learned that the Australian government had bought an anti-Rh product from Canada to use during the shortage.

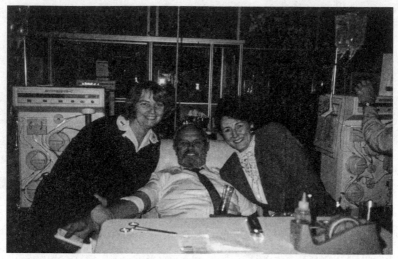

Left to right: Lizzie Thyne, James Harrison, and Robyn Barlow.

Robyn marched into the director's office and said, "James's daughter is about to have another baby, and she has to have *his product.*"

Dr. Archer understood, and said, "Of course she should have her father's anti-D."

"It's the right thing to do, considering James's service to his country," Robyn said. "Now it is just a matter of finding what is left."

Robyn phoned Tracey and instructed her, "Right after you've had the baby, sign nothing, agree to nothing, and call me. I will get you your dad's anti-D. You need the Australian product, not a foreign product. Your dad was in every batch ever made. You're his little girl. This is how he wants to protect you."

Now Robyn just needed to track down a vial that was 100 percent Australian and large parts James Harrison. James had donated from the start of the Rh program. Because he was the most consistent donor in the program in Australia, his antibodies were used in every batch ever made.

On May 21, 1995, Tracey and Andrew's second son, Scott, was born in Sydney. The proud grandparents were soon bedside, and James said the latest family member looked like a spitting image of himself. "In other words, he's a handsome devil," James said, proudly holding his eight-pound, fourteen-ounce grandson.

Tracey did as she was instructed and called Robyn at the blood bank.

Robyn didn't let on that she was worried, given she hadn't been able to find the Australian-only anti-D. She was running out of time.

She went one more time into the cold room of the blood bank. She had searched here before. But she would search again. Opening the fridge, she couldn't believe her eyes. There before her, front and center on the shelf, was one vial of anti-D. *How in the world did I miss this?* she wondered, grabbing it off the shelf. She headed to the back office staff, and said she needed it sent right away to the hospital. There were a few nods, but no one moved. "We have a VIP mom waiting for it," she tried again.

Finally, when she still got little response, she said, "It's for James's daughter. *Our James!*" At that, everyone stood up. In record time, they had it packed and were heading out the door. They would hand-deliver it—straight to the hospital, and straight into Tracey's doctor's hands. Even here, in the back office, James was a star. Even more than that, he was one of their own.

CHAPTER NINETEEN
The Mother of Invention

On the evening of September 10, 2001, a series of ominous thunderstorms rumbled through New York City, while Hurricane Erin loomed dangerously a few hundred miles off the Eastern seaboard. The unsettled weather conditions convinced John Gorman to change his flight back to San Diego to the next morning.

With extra time on his hands, John decided to have dinner that night in Midtown Manhattan with his son, Cito, daughter Alex, and Cito's fiancée, Emma. John was now officially retired from blood banking at Columbia and New York University, though he was busier than ever with his East Coast consulting work and his various inventions—some of which had by now earned him millions of dollars. It had been more than three decades since his groundbreaking Rh discovery, but from his new home base in California, John was keeping his finger on the pulse of the latest Rh research.

At the Midtown restaurant, John greeted Cito, who was working for a small company, Pachyderm Consulting, doing computer and network setup for corporate clients and nonprofits. Cito had a job at the World Trade Center at nine A.M. the next morning.

As dinner commenced, the chat around the table turned to whether businessman Michael Bloomberg would win the Republican nomination in the New York mayoral primary the next day. Alex, who had graduated from Amherst College, talked about her job in the epidemiology and statistics division of the American Lung Association in New York. John, for his part, was fixated on his AI word project, having made progress programming his computer to be more like Hal of *2001: A Space Odyssey.*

"I know exactly how sentences are parsed," John said at dinner. "I can now throw very complicated sentences at the computer and it knows the synaptic tree." Cito continued to work closely with his dad on the Words Project.

After dinner, the Gormans parted ways late on what continued to be a stormy night. Back at his hotel, John managed a few hours of sleep before heading to Kennedy airport for a seven A.M. flight on a new airline, JetBlue. The storms had passed through, replaced with cloudless blue skies and sunshine. Hurricane Erin was no longer threatening to make landfall. *Great day to fly,* John thought, settling into his plane seat. Shades were drawn all around him. Everyone appeared to be intent on sleeping.

A few hours into his trip to California, John turned on the inflight television. The image onscreen made no sense. *What is this?* John got his glasses out to get a better look. Smoke was pouring out of a gaping hole in the upper floors of the North Tower of the World Trade Center. John read the words, "BREAKING NEWS: Capitol, Treasury, White House evacuated." He grabbed some headphones. More breaking news: "World Trade Center Disaster." The newscaster recounted what had just happened: A plane had flown into the North Tower at 8:46 A.M. Another plane slammed into the South Tower at 9:03 A.M. John stared at the screen. "BREAKING NEWS: Both Towers at WTC Collapse."

His eyes filled with tears. *Cito. My God. Cito is there.*

John wasn't the only one tuning in. Call buttons for flight attendants lit up. Passengers frantically dug into purses and bags for their cell phones, but no one had a connection. *Cito is always on time.* John stared at the screen. "BREAKING NEWS: America Under Attack." The JetBlue pilot came on with an announcement. The Federal

Aviation Administration had ordered all civilian planes in U.S. airspace grounded, immediately. The pilot said there were several thousand planes, including this one, being diverted. Their airliner was to land in Wichita, Kansas. John put his head in his hands.

John could only sit and wait. *Was Cito there?* Images of the collapsing towers filled the screens. People trapped inside leapt to their deaths.

Cito had left his home in the Williamsburg neighborhood of Brooklyn early, hopping on the L train to Union Square, then caught the train downtown to Bowling Green, about a ten-minute walk to the World Trade Center. He looked at his watch and picked up the pace. Taking the stairs of the subway two at a time, he reached the street. He stopped in his tracks. People were staring up at the sky, and many were crying. White paper streamed through the air.

Cito saw the smoke. The World Trade Center.

He checked at his watch. His start time at the World Trade Center had been moved back to 9:30. His dad should have departed Kennedy hours earlier. Cito fished in his bag for his cell phone. No reception.

The morning sky had turned dark. Sudden rumbles sent people sprinting for cover. Cito ran with a crowd into the lobby of a building. People were already packed in like sardines.

There was another rumble and people started running again. Clutching his heavy laptop, Cito ran, too, making his way uptown. His mom, Carol, lived on West Sixty-Third Street. He would head there.

Walking north, he paused at Eighteenth Street along the Hudson River. Looking downtown, he saw massive clouds of billowing smoke. The Twin Towers were *gone.*

Cito stopped at a fire station at Thirty-Second Street and asked whether he could donate blood. He wanted to do something, anything. He was told to come back later. He walked for what felt like hours. Finally, he made it to his mom's apartment. Carol took one look at her son, sweaty and covered in ash, and burst into tears. She reassured

Cito that his fiancée, Emma, was safe. Emma also had stopped at a fire station to try to donate blood.

John landed in Wichita, still not sure whether his son was dead or alive. Finally, his cell phone had reception. Within seconds, a call came in from Julia in San Diego. "Cito is safe," she said. "Everyone is okay." Now it was John's turn to break down.

Three days later, John was able to fly from Wichita to San Diego. He had sought out every newspaper that Wichita had to offer and listened as President Bush vowed to extract punishment for the "evil" acts. Like Americans everywhere, John remained glued to the news. As soon as he could, he checked in with former blood bank colleagues in New York. He was impressed that more than fifty-two thousand people had donated blood to the New York Blood Center in the days after September 11. Everyone—Cito and Emma included—had felt desperate to contribute something positive. Across the United States, blood centers saw a similarly striking surge in donations, collecting close to six hundred thousand more units in the fall of 2001 than they would usually—marking the largest blood donation surge in history. There were lines to donate blood at American Red Cross blood banks. Nearly every member of Congress in Washington was photographed donating blood.

Having spent more than forty years in blood banks, John knew that war always prompted a surge in donations and was in fact what started the very first national blood collection program in the United States. In anticipation of a second world war, the Red Cross began a national program to collect blood for the U.S. military. Dried plasma was used to treat soldiers during World War II. Blood donations multiplied again during the Korean War. The focus on donating blood was a small silver lining to a horrific ongoing tragedy. While 60 percent of the American adult population was eligible to donate blood, only 5 percent of those eligible did so regularly.

Arriving home in Del Mar, a seaside town in San Diego, John settled into his downstairs office, with multiple computer screens and a few decades' worth of files, many on Rh research, trials, and stories. John would always love Manhattan—it was where he had made his American dream come true—but it had for several years felt more like a hassle than a thrill. He had loved his New York flat on the thirty-ninth floor, but didn't love what awaited him outside: traffic, noise, and the challenges of just getting around. He had also started to believe that Manhattan was the number one target for terrorist attacks, even telling Julia a year earlier, "They're going to bomb Manhattan for sure." The two had decided, when the time was right, to find "the best place in the country to live." They looked at houses in Portland, Oregon; San Francisco, California; Chesapeake Bay, Maryland; and South Carolina. But they always returned to New York feeling they hadn't seen anything better than what they already had. Then one day John saw an ad in the *Wall Street Journal* for what looked like a beautiful home a block from the beach in Del Mar, California. "Let's go look at this one," John said. He and Julia did so, and it was love at first sight.

John continued to churn out new ideas while still returning to unresolved theories of his past. He had followed the development of a theory he'd first articulated in 1960 around the existence of "benign cells" in an immune system. John believed before anyone else in the medical establishment that tolerance was "an active immune response." He wrote of "lymphocytes that were immunologically incompetent or tolerant cells that didn't harm you." But his belief that benign cells had to exist to explain immunological tolerance was dismissed.

For four years, John had evangelized about these benign cells wherever he went, from Columbia and Melbourne to Boston, Stanford, and Oxford. He shared his theory with researchers, professors, and editors at dinner parties, conferences, and blood bank meetings. He felt as passionately about this idea as he had about Rh. After finally getting a paper published on his suppressor cell theory in the journal *Blood* in 1964, he still got no traction, and eventually gave up pushing the idea.

Sitting at his desk in Del Mar, he remained intrigued by the difference between ideas embraced and ideas rejected. Apparently, there had been a researcher in Canada who had come up with the idea for using passive antibodies to treat Rh disease years before John had landed on the idea. But the Canadian's ideas never gained traction.

John's theories around tolerance as an active immune response was picked up a decade later by researchers at Yale. In the 1970s, John read the published findings of Yale researcher Dick Gershon, who independently published his own "suppressor cell" theory that tolerance was an active process rather than deletion, a theory that was almost identical to his own. John had been at a dinner at the home of Columbia's pathology chairman discussing the theory with Gershon.

Unlike John's proposal, which did not take hold at all among immunologists, to his great disappointment, Gershon's "suppressor cell" was widely noted and stimulated an enormous amount of research over the next few years, producing controversial findings. The research was eventually dropped. Fortunately, however, Gershon's idea that immunological tolerance was an active immune response was pursued relentlessly from 1982 on by Japanese researcher and immunologist Shimon Sakaguchi, who performed the definitive experiments in 1995, specifically identifying and characterizing the subpopulation of regulatory T cells, or "Treg cells," that suppress autoimmune responses. He showed that the removal of these specifically identified Treg cells from healthy animals elicited the spontaneous development of a spectrum of autoimmune diseases. When Sakaguchi restored the cells, the animals recovered. He claimed, much as John had asserted decades earlier, that "without these cells the body would attack healthy cells." The Treg cells—which didn't have a name when John was writing about them—acted as a check to prevent autoimmune reactions. Like John,

Sakaguchi was labeled something of a dreamer at first. But Sakaguchi persevered with his research until he discovered that the FoxP3 molecule was essential in the regulatory T cells and later found the genes that regulate T cell development. As his work was confirmed many times, Sakaguchi would be credited as the discoverer of the T-reg cell—and hyped as a Nobel Prize contender.

It was a reminder to John that inventions and breakthroughs are seldom a solitary success, and sometimes took decades. Scientists still remained puzzled over exactly how passive antibodies work to prevent Rh disease.

He had come to believe more in the multiplicity of discovery than in any solitary approach. History was rife with discoveries that were simultaneous—including the breakthrough around Rh disease. He could think of dozens of inventions that were discovered simultaneously, whether the system of calculus by Isaac Newton and Gottfried Wilhelm Leibniz or the theory on the evolution of the species by Charles Darwin and Alfred Russel Wallace. The same went for artists, musicians, even novelists who wrote stories with the same core themes but created them on separate continents, independent of one another. Weren't inventions just a response to the world around them? And what would that world look like if heroic people from all walks of life didn't step forward?

CHAPTER TWENTY
Golden Arm, Broken Heart

The records began to pile up, surpassing the bromeliads in James Harrison's backyard, the wine and port collection that had taken over a part of his house, and the pug figurines that filled his living room shelves. Five hundred donations of blood as of June 1991, six hundred donations as of June 1995, seven hundred donations as of April 1999.

With the milestones came parties organized by Robyn Barlow and Nurse Lizzie, complete with cakes made by donor Olive Semmler and her daughter, Val. James received badges and plaques, and paeans in verse, song, toasts, and roasts. Then came the news stories on James, first in Red Cross publications, then in small local papers and community newsletters, and eventually in major Australian dailies.

"Worth Bottling" read the headline when James made his 537th donation. "He Chases Blood Donor Record" read another headline when James reached 600 donations. A photo showed him smiling and holding a bag of his plasma, the straw-colored liquid containing the all-important anti-Rh antibodies. Stories not only detailed the successes of the Rh program—one million doses of anti-Rh made for women in need by donors—but also the challenges: "Australia is currently facing a critical shortage of plasma." Another story, pegged to James's 613th donation, was titled "Plasma Prince!" and lauded his donation of "an awesome 367.8 liters of blood," including antibodies that had saved his own grandson, Scott. Another headline read: "Walking Blood Bank Saves Babies' Lives."

In June 1999—at 705 donations—James received word that he was the recipient of an Order of Australia medal for service to his community, a tribute that came with a letter detailing the "approval of Her Majesty Queen Elizabeth the Second, Queen of Australia and Sovereign of the Order of Australia."

Now, in June 2003, James, who was sixty-six, and his wife, Barb, were invited to a swanky event in a ballroom in north Sydney for another award, one that particularly appealed to James. Seated at their table was Jane Flemming, an Australian Olympic track and field athlete and former Commonwealth Games gold medalist. Other notables and award recipients shared tables with journalists, television newscasters, and local officials.

When James's name was called, Barb squeezed his hand and watched him make his way to the stage. She had recently become a plasma donor herself. It felt to her like ten donations was a lot: getting there, waiting, donating, resting, getting home. For James, though, it was just a part of his routine. After nearly forty-five years of marriage, Barb knew better than anyone that when James committed to something, that was that. He had never missed a single dinner meeting of the Apex Club in over twenty-two years. Being stubborn served him well.

Onstage, the emcee made the announcement: "James Harrison, you are here because you have been successful in setting . . . a new Guinness World Record!" James smiled and nodded. After all these years of donating, he still didn't know what the fuss was about. The emcee waited for the applause to settle.

"You have donated blood *eight hundred and eight times*! That is *one thousand seventy-seven* units of blood! James, you have made it into the *Guinness Book of Records* for the most blood donated by a single person." A medal on a ribbon was hung around his neck, and James was photographed holding a framed certificate and a magnum of wine to add to his collection.

The emcee noted that 17 percent of mothers in Australia were at risk of Rh disease, but there were fewer than two hundred donors in the country's Rh program.

"Details of your record have been entered into our record books," the host said. "You made your 808th blood donation on May 19, 2003. Welcome to the select band of Guinness World Records. You are the Man with the Golden Arm!"

James received a standing ovation.

He was deeply humbled. "All I've done is donate each fortnight," he told the crowd. "I started when I was eighteen. There are many other dedicated donors besides me. No one donates for money—there's no money in it in Australia. I donate because it is necessary to keep people alive, to give our babies a chance at life. I donate because of what others get out of it."

He urged attendees to "give an hour of your time to save a life." Before exiting the stage, he held up the award and said, "This is a record I'd like to see broken, because that would mean someone will donate even more blood."

As James and Barb left the event, James was stopped and thanked again and again. One woman surprised James by hugging him and breaking into tears. "I've had seven babies thanks to you," she said, pulling out her wallet to share photos of her kids.

James was unusually quiet on the way home, replaying what the woman had said. He had known, of course, that his plasma was being used to help parents have healthy babies. But this felt different. It was the same feeling he had when Tracey needed anti-D to protect Scott. It was this direct link to a life, a hand extended and accepted. He had seen the woman's photos of her sons and daughters, her boy at the piano, her daughter doing ballet, another boy playing cricket, another jumping into a lake. It dawned on him: The gift was as much his as it was hers. Her gift was babies. Her gift was family. His gift was meeting someone whose life was so much better because of something simple he had done. Anti-D was the only way that some couples could have healthy children. It was the one card they had to play.

Barb couldn't resist ribbing James a bit, saying she'd now have to get used to living with a celebrity.

"Oh, sure—my fifteen minutes of fame," James said.

Barb and James had begun to synchronize their blood donations, going to the Sydney blood bank together and stopping for coffee or ice cream afterward. Barb had just signed on to become a donor in the Rh project and was getting her Rh-negative blood boosted with Rh-positive blood. She was told that it could take up to six months for the boosting to work. Tracey was hardly surprised when she learned that her mum was now a donor in the Rh program as well. Donating blood was what the Harrisons did, starting with her grandfather Reginald. For as long as Tracey could remember, Friday always meant someone was making a trip to the blood bank.

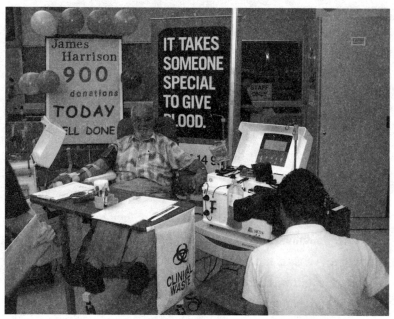

James Harrison continues to reach milestones in donating blood.

Back home, James found a place on their crowded shelves for his Guinness World Records plaque and medal. Both retired, James and Barb settled in to plan their next caravan in the RV to another far-flung corner of Australia. This was their time to do whatever they wanted.

As soon as the RV was packed, they headed out on their drive to the Barossa Valley, a renowned wine region northeast of Adelaide in southern Australia. They could take their time to enjoy the views from the Great Ocean Road along the southeastern coast. The winding road was commissioned in 1919 to honor those who had lost their lives in World War I. Thousands of servicemen built the road by hand in the years after the war.

Driving along the coastline, James and Barb saw surfers riding massive waves. They stopped for a bite to eat in charming small towns, where there were craft fairs and farmers markets. They toured inland through national parks and delighted in seeing southern koala bears, with fur that was more brown than gray like their northern counterparts.

They held hands as they watched the sunset that turned the rock formations known as the Twelve Apostles off the shore of Port Campbell National Park into changing canvases of red, terra-cotta, beige, and sandstone. The waves and wind of the Southern Ocean were eroding the limestone stacks, which jutted nearly 150 feet high. James and Barb imagined the peril faced by sailors and seafarers who had to navigate the treacherous passage where the Bass Strait and Southern Ocean met.

"Why in the world is it called the Twelve Apostles when there are only nine rocks?" Barb asked. James laughed and said it used to be called something like "the sow and the piglets."

They found caravan parks for the night and enjoyed wine and their own cooking. They'd head out the next day, stopping in more towns, watching the stirred-up surf, and taking photos of the occasional rainbow.

They shared stories that made them laugh, including the RV trip when James decided to buy several cases of 1967 port to mark Tracey's birth year. He had figured he would open it for her and her friends on her twenty-first birthday. "But then Tracey's birthday comes around, and I was like, 'I'm not wasting hundred-dollar bottles of port on these hoodlum friends!'" Barb reminded him of another trip to a wine region when he'd insisted on buying *thirty-two cases* of wine and port to bring home, leaving them with barely enough room to walk or sleep in the RV.

Each night, they returned to one of James's favorite sayings: "This is the good life."

They always kept a lookout for one spot decidedly off the tourist path. They would visit any blood bank or donor mobile and ask whether they could donate.

James would inevitably get: "Oh, you're the Man with the Golden Arm!" from nurses or donors. Several people asked to have their pictures taken with him.

Barb just shook her head. *He's getting more than his fifteen minutes*, she thought.

They both had worked, saved, and lived modestly to do just this: enjoy their golden years. James had left his job at the railway before Barb retired from teaching. She was at Doonside High School for twenty-five years. James was surprised that he loved being the house husband, as he called it, doing the grocery shopping, ironing, gardening, and light cleaning. He left the cooking to the expert, Barb. When Tracey and her family visited, they were struck by how her parents took care of one another, and how Barb doted on James. The two had recently moved into their new home in Umina Beach, leaving Tracey and Andrew and their boys with the home in Doonside, about an hour's drive from Sydney and ninety minutes to Umina Beach. The weather was milder and warmer in Umina Beach, and James and Barb's new neighborhood was quiet. There was a lawn bowling club about a block away, complete with several restaurants inside the complex. Barb and James only occasionally returned to Junee, their old hometown, to visit their parents' graves. James's mom, Peggy, had died in 1995, and Reginald in 1997.

Overall, James and Barb had never been happier than they were in retirement. They kept busy with chores around the house, new recipes, and attending various club meetings. And, of course, they made regular trips to Sydney to donate blood and see the grandkids. But they were always eager to hit the road again in search of their next adventure.

In March of 2003, Barb and James headed out with their caravan club to the northern beaches of Sydney. They had about twenty RVs in their club, and James was club president. It was the beginning of autumn in Australia, when the weather was predictably nice, never too warm or too cold. They visited different beaches by day and pulled into caravan parks late afternoons, setting up their awnings, tables, and chairs, preparing food, and opening bottles of wine.

At the end of the long weekend, James and Barb agreed to join friends for a walk on the beach. As they headed down a grassy knoll, Barb slipped on the wet grass and took a spill down an embankment.

"My ankle!" she cried out. When James got to her, he took one look at her ankle and yelled out, "Call an ambulance." It was bad. Barb's foot was pointing the wrong way.

The closest medical facility was the Mona Vale Hospital on the Pittwater peninsula between Manly and Palm Beach. That's where James and Barb would have to go. Once there, Barb was told that she needed surgery to put plates in her ankle.

After the surgery, Barb spent four days in the hospital. In James's mind, that was about three days too long. On day one, James had concluded that this was a hospital they needed to get out of as fast as possible. It was understaffed, the food was inedible, and even basic supplies were hard to come by. He heard of emergency room patients being bumped for five days. He had heard talk of other hospitals across New

South Wales being closed because of budgetary cutbacks. Elective surgery was being halted for a three-week period as a cost-cutting measure. It felt like Mona Vale was days away from being closed permanently.

"We need to get you out of here as soon as possible," James said to Barb at the hospital. When they finally found a doctor to discharge them, there were no wheelchairs to be found. Barb's foot was in a cast. The nursing staff didn't know whether there were any wheelchairs on the premises.

"This is a hospital," James protested. "You don't have wheelchairs?"

"I'll find one," James said, finally heading off on a search. He returned about thirty minutes later. There was apparently one wheelchair in the entire hospital. Barb was released with no medication and no postoperative home-care instructions.

Barb had always taken care of James, but now it was James's turn to care for Barb. Once home from the hospital, she still insisted on cooking, and managed to do so hobbling about on crutches, her foot in a cast. The kitchen in their Umina Beach residence was her favorite room in the house and had been built to her specifications. But James was concerned. He could see that she was struggling. Short of breath and in discomfort, Barb insisted she was fine.

When Tracey called on the evening of March 31, about two weeks after her mom had been released from the hospital, she, too, was surprised to hear her mom short of breath. Still, Barb delighted in hearing the boys—Jarrod was twelve, and Scott was nine—play in the background. Then Barb started coughing and wheezing again. She told Tracey not to worry.

The next morning, James was up early making coffee. He heard that Barb was up. It sounded like she was in the bathroom washing her face.

"I'm making coffee," he offered.

No reply.

"Love, do you want coffee?" he asked again.

Then he heard an anguished cry: "Jim!" There was a terrible crash. He ran to the bathroom.

Barb was on the floor. Her head was bleeding. She must have hit her head on the chair on the way down. Blood pooled under her head. He felt for her pulse. "Barb!" He started CPR.

"Barb, I'm here," he said desperately.

Nothing.

"Barb!" he cried, holding her shoulders.

"Barb!"

He tried mouth to mouth again.

"Barb, I'm right here," James said.

He tried again. Nothing. He held his wife.

Barb was gone.

His hands shaking, James put a towel under Barb's head. He ran to the kitchen to call 911.

He didn't know how to make the next call. *What do you say?* Slowly, he dialed Tracey. *How do I say this?*

She answered on the second ring.

"I'm getting the kids off to school," Tracey said, sounding harried.

"Your mother has died," James said.

Tracey said, "Right, Dad. April Fool's! Weird joke!" It was April 1, 2005.

There was silence.

"Dad?"

"Tracey," James said again, this time slower. "Your mother has died."

Tracey stopped. She motioned to her husband, Andrew.

"What are you talking about?" she asked.

"Your mother hit her head. She died. This morning. Just now."

Her dad's voice was detached. Far away.

"Dad, we're on our way," she said. Tracey and Andrew got into the car with the boys, called the school, and headed to Umina Beach. It was the longest ninety minutes of her life. Arriving at the house, Tracey saw that the ambulance and coroner were there.

"Why don't you take the boys somewhere while I go in?" she said to Andrew.

Tracey walked in tentatively. Seeing her dad, she began to cry.

"Do you want to see her?" James asked, nodding toward the bathroom.

"Yes," Tracey said. But she approached the hallway, she turned back. She didn't want to see her mum like that.

Tracey sat down on the sofa next to her dad. The coroner said he would be removing the body. Tracey could see that her dad was on autopilot. He was making sense, but his voice wasn't his own. He talked about needing to make funeral arrangements and how he should call some funeral homes.

Then he looked at Tracey and said, "She was just here. Now she is gone."

In the days that followed, James and Tracey were told that Barb had died of a blood clot, possibly two clots, one to the heart and one to the lungs. She was sixty-six years old.

Medical personnel in the coroner's office asked James whether Barb was on any blood thinner. No. Did she wear compression stockings after surgery? No. "Nothing," James said. They had been given nothing when they left the hospital.

After Barb's death, James sat for hours, alone on his sofa. Family and friends visited and brought food and casseroles. Tracey tried to teach her dad how to use the oven, stove, and microwave. This had always been her mom's domain.

"Call me each morning to see if I'm still alive," James instructed Tracey. He didn't know how to live without Barb.

Days passed without James turning a light on in the house. He sat alone with his memories. The Barb of his childhood was the brave farmer's daughter who rode her pony to school. Barb as a young woman took his breath away when she stood on the platform at the train station. He thought of their wedding, their starter house with the thirty-two tree stumps. He could see Barb so clearly in the kitchen, smiling and waving as she made him lemonade. He thought of the rugby matches they went to in their station wagon, always bringing the pugs and dressing them in the blue and gold of their favorite team. He thought of Tracey as a baby, and how happy he and Barb were to have a daughter. He remembered how Barb had made a sandwich for him every day for work. They played cards with friends every Saturday night, just as their parents had done. Barb was the one person who had always looked after him, from his days as a sickly youth to standing by his side as an adult. She never stopped telling him: "James, you are a beautiful man."

Their golden years were ahead of them.

James remained entrenched on the couch, the light of day changing, the weather growing colder. His stamp collection stayed unopened. Dishes piled up in the sink. Tracey called to check on him every morning.

His life had been about giving blood—giving life. Now it was blood that had taken the one he loved the most.

He called Robyn at the blood bank.

"Barb has died," he told her. "I won't be in to donate."

CHAPTER TWENTY-ONE
Peace in the Azaleas

One by one, they made their way to the altar of the church. At the altar, friends and family sprinkled flower petals on top of the closed casket. Final words were offered. Tears flowed. By the procession's end, the mahogany casket was blanketed in brightly hued petals. The flowers were azaleas—Barb's favorite.

"Barb would have been surprised," James thought, sitting in the front row of the church in Palmdale, a suburb of Sydney, watching the outpouring of love and warmth. He had expected about eighty people at the funeral, as he hadn't had the energy to do much inviting. But the church was standing room only, with close to two hundred people. They were there to celebrate the life of Barbara Harrison, wife of James, mother of Tracey, and grandmother of Jarrod and Scott—the family matriarch who had died the morning of April 1, 2005, at age sixty-six. There were teachers from Barb's school, nurses and staff from the Red Cross, James's former colleagues from the railway, friends from their various clubs, and family young and old.

James had asked his brother-in-law, Ken Thrift, to deliver the eulogy, fearing he would not be able to stay composed when called on to tell the story of Barb. Ken was married to James's sister Margaret and was a police commissioner comfortable with public speaking. He had adored Barb.

Standing at the altar, Ken began in a commanding voice: "I regarded Barbara as my sister, not my sister-in-law. That's how close we were."

He recounted their happy times together during caravans around Australia, learning about wine, volunteering, and simply sharing their lives.

"We had a lot of fun together," Ken continued. "I loved Barbara. I had four brothers, and never had a sister—until Barbara. She was a country girl, of course. I was a country boy. In that way, we both regarded ourselves as outlaws. But Barbara was always thinking of others."

Margaret was seated with her three children, Kylie, Danielle, and Richard, now ages thirty-nine, forty-one, and forty-three. The older two had been protected by James's anti-D when the shots first became available. Barb had been like a sister to Margaret, too, and her death was devastating. Margaret would never forget the morning of April 1, when James called in a monotone to deliver the news. She was on the phone with her daughter, and Ken had answered their home phone. She watched Ken's expression change quickly. Margaret told her daughter: "Wait a minute. Dad is talking with Uncle Jim." Ken came to her and said, "You better sit down. Barbara has died. This morning. Instantly."

The funeral was delayed for weeks while the coroner did an inquest, which concluded that Barb had died from two blood clots—one to the heart, one to the lungs. When Margaret and Ken made it to James's house in Umina Beach the day Barb had passed away, all James could say was, "How could she leave?"

Margaret could see that James was on autopilot, thanking people for coming, listening to stories, and accepting condolences. He was pleased he had hired a group of women funeral directors called the White Ladies, and was sure that Barb would have liked that. The White Ladies were impeccable in their white skirt suits and red fedoras.

Tracey and Andrew and their boys Jarrod and Scott sat in the front row. Tracey watched the long procession and feared they were going to run out of azaleas. Her dad had picked the flowers himself from their garden, but no one anticipated this many people. Scott, who was ten, was hit particularly hard by the loss; it was his first death. Scott always looked forward to his time in the kitchen with grandma. She taught him the proper way to cut up fruits and vegetables, the best way to mix, whisk, and blend various concoctions, and her techniques for preparing different dishes. They made macaroons and always had a hard time waiting for them to cool before sampling them. The three generations of Harrisons took walks around the neighborhood or headed to the beach for the afternoon. Most nights before dinner, Scott and grandma picked flowers from the garden. "We'll decorate the table with our flowers," she told him.

Ken ended the eulogy, and the minister approached to offer final prayers and hymns. The time had come for the coffin to be carried out by the White Ladies, three women on each side. James was not prepared to watch the casket go. Tracey had seen her dad cry only once before— at the funeral of her granddad, his father, Reginald, about eight years earlier. Barb was going to be cremated, a wish that she and James had discussed long before. James watched the casket leave the church and knew he now would never see her again.

Earlier in the day, before the public service, James, Tracey, Margaret, and Ken had time alone with Barb, open casket. Tracey had picked a favorite outfit for Barb's burial clothes. She fixed Barb's hair the way she thought her mom would like it. Standing before her mom's open casket that day, Tracey placed a rose inside the coffin. She wished they'd had more time together, quietly telling her mom, "If we had one more day, I would want to spend the whole day talking." Tracey knew now she had made the mistake of thinking, "We'll talk later." Later was this. She looked back on her days when she and her dad—the two shared an offbeat sense of humor—would have fun needling Barb. Her mother was good-natured about it, but Tracey wondered whether she had told her she loved her as much as she should have. Probably not.

At the wake that followed the funeral, more stories were shared. "Even some of Tracey's friends made the drive," James remarked. He held it together, listening to memories of Barb as a friend and Barb as a teacher. He was doing okay, staying strong—until the music began to play. Track by track, he listened to a playlist of their favorite country songs. Hearing Slim Dusty's "Waltzing Matilda" sent James in search of a chair and a private moment to himself. The lyrics always got him: "You'll come a-waltzing, you scoundrel, with me." Barb was his waltz. He was her scoundrel. He didn't know who he was without Barb. He'd met her the day she was born, when he was two-and-a-half years old and his parents said they were all going to the hospital to meet the new Lindbeck baby, a girl. He never imagined he'd be a widower. He had figured he would go first.

James arrived back at his home in Umina Beach exhausted. The lights were out, and the house was quiet. Scenes from the day played over in his mind. He was worried about Tracey. When he'd asked Tracey to call him every morning to make sure he was still alive, he was sincere. He needed checking on. But he had a secret agenda, too, which was to check on Tracey. She was looking after him, but he was looking after her. Whenever Tracey visited him, she kept searching for certain missing recipes. The macaroon recipe was nowhere to be found. Tracey couldn't understand where it could possibly have gone. James knew that the recipes were about more than cooking. They were another way for Tracey to hold on to her mom.

He went to the kitchen to make a pot of tea. Before Barb died, he'd never even boiled water. Tracey had to teach him. The weeks that followed the funeral were like those preceding it. He read instructions on how to heat food, opened Barb's mail, and took calls from people just hearing the news. He went for days without seeing anyone. Trips to the doctor became his connection to the outside world.

One day, his doctor asked him whether he had any hobbies.

James smiled. "When I was five, I was given a packet of stamps and a small stamp album that I put them in," he said. "My relatives would buy stamps for me or give me money to buy stamps. Over the years, I've collected over one hundred thousand stamps in more than forty albums."

"Are you still collecting?" the doctor asked.

"Not now," James said.

"Start again," the doctor said bluntly. "I want you to do something to stop the depression."

Back home, James thought about the doctor's advice. He had given up adding to his stamp collection months earlier because he and Barb were on the road, busy with their new adventures in retirement. Sitting on the sofa, the TV on, he calculated he was spending $105 a month on his cable bill. After a few hours of mulling it over, he decided he would cancel his cable service. Instead he would spend the $105 a month collecting stamps again.

His doctor, hearing the news a few weeks later, said: "It's a good start."

James began adding stamps from Great Britain and America. The images were gorgeous and high quality. Collecting made him want to share his new treasures, something that was always part of the fun. A few weeks later, he returned to his stamp-collecting group, and appreciated that his friends were happy to see him. Then his caravan club came calling. After James demurred, saying he wasn't ready to travel, his friends told him he was coming on the next trip. They refused to take no for an answer. A few hours into the first trip without Barb, James was sure he had made a big mistake. Barb's seat in the RV was empty, and he kept wanting to talk to her, to point out funny names of towns,

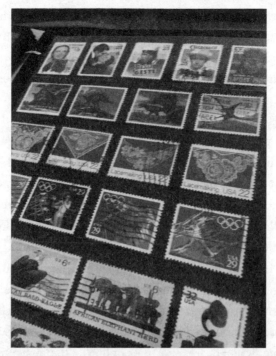

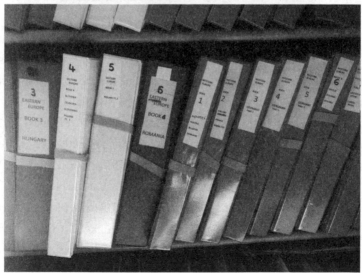

James Harrison turned back to his stamp collection to alleviate his grief over the loss of his wife.

to hear her talk about the scenery and wildlife. But when the caravan club stopped for a meal, James found himself surrounded. The caravan crew brought over food and chairs and settled in. Being with people again was nice. Before he knew it, he was agreeing to join them on trips to Perth, Queensland, and back to the Barossa Valley.

He was even learning to cook a few basic dishes. He had told himself, "You either got to eat or die, so you better learn to cook."

James had a more complicated relationship with blood. The coroner's report was never far from his mind. Blood clots had ended Barb's life. He had replayed the weeks before her death a thousand times: the fall down the grassy slope, the operation, the understaffed hospital, the lack of home-care instructions. He second-guessed everything that had happened. If only he had been holding her arm as they walked. If only he had taken her to another hospital. If only they had gone to see her doctor upon returning from the Mona Vale hospital. If only he had inquired more about medication to prevent clotting or asked more questions about any warning signs. She had shortness of breath, but he figured it was a normal part of her recovery. Her death seemed entirely preventable.

But when he went to these dark places, he would think about donors like Olive Semmler, who had continued to give blood despite losing so many babies to Rh disease. Her kindness, in the face of tragedy, had always inspired him. And for James, there was also the miracle of blood itself. Blood had saved his life. His blood had saved lives. It had a dual nature. James looked at the veins in his arms and thought, "But isn't that life itself? You got to take the good with the bad."

On the day Barb died, James had called Robyn at the blood bank in Sydney to say he wasn't going to be coming in to donate blood. He was in shock. Barb was there one minute, gone the next. He needed time to find his balance. Though he now accepted that he wouldn't find his balance again anytime soon, donating blood was who he was. It was one thing that didn't have to change because Barb died.

The next week, James was back at the blood bank. He knew if Barb were watching, she would be happy.

When James walked into the Red Cross center, Robyn and Nurse Lizzie welcomed him. Robyn hugged James tightly.

"We are happy to see you," she said.

"I'm happy to be here," James said. The blood bank had changed over the years—it was a more bureaucratic place—but James still considered it his home away from home.

Robyn hadn't been able to attend Barb's funeral, as she was recovering from surgery and at the same time was caring for her mother, who was facing end-of-life struggles and had been moved into a nursing facility. Robyn had been divorced for some time from the pilot who had gone off to the Vietnam War—his departure prompting her to take the job at the Red Cross—and she was now living with a pioneering hematologist, Dr. Harry Kronenberg.

Robyn had been devastated to hear of Barb's tragic passing. She grieved for James, and she also lamented the loss of Barb as a donor. Robyn had just found out that Barb's last blood test showed she was successfully immunized to join the Rh program. Barb, too, was producing anti-D that could be harvested to protect babies. Robyn had excitedly told the blood bank director: "Won't it be wonderful to see husband and wife donating together?"

James was touched by the kindness of everyone he saw at the blood bank that day. He told Robyn, "I've decided that I'll give up donating blood when the nurse has to use two hands to get the needle in." Robyn laughed, but she knew that James was serious.

Robyn returned to her desk. She had spared James stories of her own travails, as well as the stories of her changing job. New regulations and world health advisories on blood collection were drowning the center in additional paperwork around precautions, ID requirements, tracking, monitoring, and follow-up. Times were certainly different from the folksy days of the past, when Nurse Lizzie could reward donors by gifting them her newly hatched chicks or Olive Semmler could hand out cookies or slices of cake. The ever-changing requirements placed a burden on the center and donors alike. Donating took longer. Donors had to be interviewed every visit, regardless of how long they had been giving blood. They had to fill out forms before giving blood and after. Eligibility criteria were changed. Records had gone from handwritten to automated to digitized, yet somehow the technological progress slowed the process down. Everything was entered into the system, right down to how many cotton swabs were used with each blood draw.

Except for the occasions when James and the other founding Rh donors came in, Robyn sometimes barely recognized the place. The blood bank had graduated from manual plasmapheresis, where nurses had to carefully squeeze packs, seal them, and run a saline line before returning the plasma to the donor. Plasmapheresis was now done by a machine, which they called their "washing machine." Whole blood was passed through a cell separator, and a centrifuge separated red blood cells, plasma, and platelets, eventually returning the red cells to the donor. The machine tracked the donor's height and weight, so the right amount of blood components was drawn. It was much more, as Robyn said, "push a button."

Over the years, Robyn, who had no formal medical training before starting at the Red Cross in the 1960s, had become an expert on blood and Rh. She had advised doctors and staff at Red Cross centers in Melbourne, Queensland, Brisbane, and Victoria on how they should set up their Rh programs. She had recently delivered a paper on Australia's pioneering hematologist and serologist Ruth Sanger—coauthor of the seminal book *Blood Groups in Man*—at an international congress of scientists and blood researchers.

But the day was coming for her to step away. And within a year, Robyn retired. Her mother, Gladys, had lived longer than anyone expected and had been happier at the nursing home than anyone predicted, but when she passed away, Robyn no longer had nursing home bills to pay. Robyn was also growing weary of the endless paperwork and regulations at the blood bank, as well as the ubiquitous talk of litigation, something that had never been a part of her job in the early years. It didn't seem possible, but she had been at the Red Cross for nearly forty years. She wanted no fanfare when she left, but promised to stay in touch and pop in for visits, as she lived just across the Sydney Harbour. She had her dream job for years and knew she was a part of a transformative medical breakthrough. She had watched up close as the treatment for Rh had fundamentally changed the health of women and their babies. She would miss the place. Before she retired, she told James, "In some ways, it's the end of who you are. It's what defines you. This has defined me. Suddenly I'm not that anymore." James understood. That's how he felt after losing Barb.

James never stopped impressing Robyn as her last day of work arrived. He was one of the few donors who never complained about the added paperwork, the new eligibility forms and waivers and disclosures. When he was handed new forms to sign, he'd say, "No problem." New photo ID required? He'd say, "Get my good side!"

James was taking the loss of Barb one day at a time. He held on to a quote he'd heard at Barb's memorial: "Grief is the price you pay for love." That made sense to him. He began accepting more invitations from the caravan club. On a trip to Queensland, the club stopped at a country music festival along the way. James was surprised when one of the musicians singled him out from the stage, saying that none other than "the Man with the Golden Arm" was in the crowd. After the concert, several women approached and thanked James for their healthy children. One woman said, "I have eight children, so I had your injection seven times."

He had kept track of his donor milestones and was always setting new goals for himself. Maybe it was the same way his dad kept adding to the neighborhoods he visited each year as Santa. James soon headed to the Sydney blood bank for another milestone. But this time, he arrived with someone near and dear—his grandson, Scott. After filling out the necessary forms—Tracey and Andrew had given permission for him to donate before the legal age of eighteen—James and Scott took their seats in side-by-side donor chairs. Scott wore a T-shirt with the Superman logo. James took a look at it and said that he should be wearing the shirt. "I'm the master and you're the apprentice," he told his grandson. James was seventy-five. Scott was sixteen. It was May 26, 2011. It was Scott's first donation, and James's one thousandth donation.

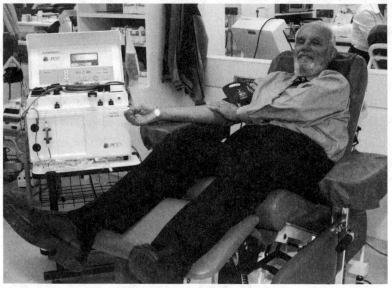

James Harrison hits another milestone—one thousand blood donations—and is joined by his grandson Scott.

James was hooked to the plasmapheresis machine, and Scott was given a red ball to squeeze. He was donating whole blood. "I always look away, even after all these years," James advised Scott.

Scott had grown up hearing about blood donations. Someone in the family always seemed to be going to the blood bank. And he had been told that his grandpa's special blood had protected him at birth. Scott had been the one to suggest that they donate blood together. "It's a great thing that you do," he told his grandpa.

Scott wasn't anxious in the slightest—until he saw the nurse approaching him with a needle bigger than he'd imagined. He took a deep breath and thought of all the good that came with giving blood.

James looked over at Scott and said, "Proud of you. Proud that we are a family of blood donors."

On the way out, James said, "Really, my thousandth donation is no more important than somebody's first donation. It costs me nothing—only time. And I have plenty of time." He hugged Scott again, watched him get on a bus, and set out for the train station.

James arrived home and put his things down on the kitchen counter before heading to the back yard. He had important news to deliver. He took a seat in his familiar chair in a familiar spot at the back of the garden, surrounded by more than forty azalea plants. This was where he came to talk to Barb. Her ashes were carefully placed in a container under an azalea in a large pot. He had told Tracey, "When I go, you put my ashes with her." So, he settled in and began to tell Barb how he had just made his one thousandth donation. "But that's not really the news," he told her. "Your grandson Scott donated with me for the first time." James told her of how Scott's eyes had grown big like saucers when he saw the size of the needle coming at him. "But he was fine. Strong. He's becoming a man." He was proud, he said, that Scott was carrying on the tradition. James stayed in the garden until the sun set. As he said goodnight, he admired the azaleas. They were all in bloom.

CHAPTER TWENTY-TWO
The Lessons of a Lifetime

John Gorman took out his iPhone and studied a map of Walwa, a small tin-mining bush town, population two hundred-sixty. The blink-or-you'll-miss-it community was where his mother, Doris, had taken her first job as a general practitioner back in the 1920s. The town of Walwa was situated about a half-mile from the Murray River on the former Murray Valley highway between Wodonga and Corryong.

John was driving in the rugged terrain of northeastern Victoria, on his way to Sydney. With John were his wife, Julia, and his younger sister, Jeanne Gorman, and her husband, Ken Allen. They were traveling to see John's brother Frank and sister-in-law Kath. John, in typical lesson mode, wanted to show Julia his childhood haunts and share his colorful family history—but it was John who was about to learn some important lessons of his own.

Before starting out on the drive, John had admired a faded photo of his mother, Doris, and father, taken in medical school in Melbourne during the early 1920s. The young students had just completed their obstetrics training and were photographed with classmates, each one holding a newborn baby. Doris was one of only a few women in her class. She and John Sr. had met when they were first-year students seated alphabetically in the lecture hall. She was Grant and he was Gorman.

After earning her medical degree, and before marrying John Sr. in 1928, Doris took the job in Walwa. She was twenty-eight years old and the only doctor for more than eighty miles in any direction. There were days when her job involved sewing up farm animals on kitchen tables—there was no vet—and other days when she'd find herself rushed to the site of the tin mine to tend to accident victims.

"I remember the story of mum having to get into the back seat of someone's car with a miner who'd been in an accident and was nearly scalped," Jeanne said during the drive. "They had to drive to the nearest town, Wodonga, where her brother was a GP. It was a good distance over terrible roads, and she was working on his head right there in the back seat. She was a brave one, wasn't she?"

Jeanne recalled, too, when she was a little girl and her mom would take her on house calls at night. "Mother would go way up in the country into the bush and walk along these dark paths with dogs barking at her to see the patients in their houses," Jeanne said. "I was terrified just sitting there in her car."

Until that moment, John had never given much thought to his mother's path being particularly brave or difficult. She was always his hard-working mom. "She was a pioneer!" Julia declared. "Brave—a heroine!"

John was struck by his wife's words, in ways that were hard to fathom. Earlier during the visit, they had stopped in Bendigo and Rochester, the towns of his childhood. John had been upset to find that the family home in Bendigo had been demolished and replaced with apartments. Still, John was able to show Julia where he'd gone to swim in the river and attended school and where he'd escaped to play hooky. Before leaving Bendigo, they had stopped at the cemetery where John and Doris were buried.

Now, in the wake of visiting his parents' graves, John wondered why he had never stopped to consider his parents' path more profoundly. Was his mother a *heroine*, as Julia said? Doris had worked as a telephone operator to put herself through medical school—surely not an easy feat—before graduating and taking the job out in the bush, where she was isolated and on her own. She practiced medicine for six decades, raised four kids, stayed married, traveled extensively by herself, and walked to her office on her last day of life, at age eighty-four.

And likewise, was his father a hero, too? During World War I, when his dad's brothers, classmates and friends were conscripted or volunteered to serve, John Sr. took a stand as a pacifist—something close to heretical in the day. Men of all ages and backgrounds were rushing to enlist. Even his teachers urged students to become soldiers. His dad read everything he could on war and on the idea of a "just war"—a concept he couldn't embrace. After much thought, he decided that he wouldn't kill, but he wouldn't sit out the war, either. He told his mother, Aggie Gorman, that he would join the war efforts as a stretcher-bearer to help the wounded. His mother, one of the few who supported his pacifism, was relieved.

John Jr. realized it must have been difficult for his father to go against the grain, to disagree with the prevailing sentiment. It takes bravery to stand up for what you believe.

As the drive to Sydney continued, John could not get the idea of heroism out of his head. He didn't disagree with Julia's use of the word for his mother, but it prompted him to think through long-held assumptions and stereotypes—and to examine his own life and legacy. Wasn't a hero someone who risked his life to save another? Heroism included valor. The hero won the battle and got the girl. A hero was George Washington, who led his battered troops across the Delaware on Christmas to surprise the British Army. A hero was a first responder who rushed toward the World Trade Center after planes flew into it on the morning of September 11. A hero like that was noble, with almost superhuman powers. Could his dad's stance of pacifism be considered heroic? His dad had been interested in the writings of Aristotle and what the philosopher terms "greatness of soul"—as defined in part as someone who helped others in need. So in this case, pacifism was about saving lives and refusing to kill. His father's life work—and his mother's—was to help others. *Wasn't that heroic in itself?*

The foursome was now headed on the next leg of their journey and would go over the Great Dividing Range before reaching Kath and Frank's home in Sydney. Julia had met Kath at John's talk in Tasmania—where Kath stole the show—and walked away thinking, "Kath could run General Motors!"

Retracing his family's steps and being tour guide to Julia made John think of his own voyage from Australia to America in 1955. The journey was long but hardly arduous—at least by comparison to what his ancestors had endured. But he, too, had left his homeland and everything he knew to seek a better life, setting sail from the port of Melbourne to chase his dreams in America.

He told Julia about being joined on the voyage by three mates from medical school: John Hamilton, Sam Breen, and Hubert de Castella. John said that Castella had a cabin in first class, but he and the others were at the back of the boat. "The way you found our cabin was you go down the stairs in the back of the ship and you make a turn toward the loudest noise. Our room was next to the engines." What he didn't tell Julia about was his fascination with the brilliant engineering of the machinery in the engine rooms.

It was John Hamilton who had managed to get the cheapest tickets he could find, returning to the port day after day to pester the ticket sellers about getting cheaper fares. Hamilton—who had labeled John "Doc" Gorman before he officially was a doctor—was always brimming with ideas. He once submitted John's bio to a television game show where contestants advanced by answering questions correctly. John was chosen for the show—and won $100. John and Hamilton were also known to skip out of medical school in Melbourne and hitchhike their way to Sydney, which they found far more exotic than Melbourne.

Their trip to America was filled with adventures along the way, too: visiting temples in Burma Rangoon; traveling through the Suez Canal; seeing Naples and Rome; renting a Volkswagen Beetle and driving around France. John had calculated that on days without stops, they were sailing west some six hundred miles and therefore were gifted an extra hour each day.

John's eyes lit up as memories about the voyage flooded back. He was also reminded of something he hadn't thought about in more than half a century, something that pleased him greatly. The barber who cut his hair onboard the ship had told him—almost smugly—that he'd go bald by the time he was forty. His hair was now gray—but he had a lot of it.

Julia, who had been unusually quiet, asked John whether his interest in heroism was his way of figuring out how to add the concept to his Words Project. But John shook his head; this was personal. He had always heralded the stories of great inventors or scientists, of leaders in war, of men who seemed imbued with extraordinary qualities. But this trip had him finding inspiration closer to home. The Gorman clan certainly had its share of characters, tinkerers, rebels, and success stories. John's great uncle Bert (Aggie's brother), had made a fortune in business in England, became politically influential, and bought a castle in Ireland, where he set up a racing stable. One of Uncle Bert's horses, a large and powerful Irish thoroughbred named Workman, won the Grand National steeplechase, England's most famous event in 1939, becoming the talk of international racing circles. In more recent times, John's cousin Hugh Niall was the chief scientist at Genentech in San Francisco, and did breakthrough research cloning and synthesizing the reproductive hormone relaxin. Hugh's sister, Brenda Niall, was an acclaimed author in Australia. Another cousin, Kevin Gorman—married to one of the most charming women John and Julia had ever met, and the son of "Uncle Dick" of Meilman Station—had nine children. Their middle son, now living in New York, was James Gorman, CEO and chairman of Morgan Stanley.

John's brother-in-law, Peter Morris, married to his younger sister Jocelyn, was knighted by the queen for his work in medicine. A towering figure in transplantation, he had devised one of the earliest tests used to match patients and donors for transplants and established the transplant program in England. Jocelyn was no slouch herself, having graduated at the top of her class from the University of Melbourne, and worked as a general practitioner in Oxford for many years. After Peter was knighted, Jocelyn became "Dame Morris."

In John's quest to eradicate Rh, he had tried to model his professional life after the great inventors and scientists like Thomas Edison, Marie Curie, and Jonas Salk, who devoted years of effort to discovering new knowledge. These were the giants he revered and had wanted to emulate. But now, John understood that heroism came from all walks of life—and that even the greatest knowledge was of no use if there was not a collective will to make the world a better place. He knew that his idea for what became the breakthrough for Rh would have ended as an idea had it not been for the dogged passion of Vince Freda and the technical skills and dedication of Bill Pollack.

John and his traveling partners were now due west of Sydney, driving through the Great Dividing Range, which ran down eastern Australia. The land was largely unspoiled, home to endangered animals and diverse flora and fauna, from bushland to forests. Once home to indigenous tribes, the area had been settled by explorers arriving in the late 1830s, at the same time the Gormans first set foot in Australia.

Finally, arriving in Sydney, everyone happily settled in for a visit with Kath and Frank. Julia, now experienced in the Gorman ways, knew she could just sit back and enjoy the exchange between the Gorman brothers. Frank was an ophthalmologist with a controversial theory around the recovery of optic nerve function through chiropractic spinal manipulation. John launched into talk of his Words Project—though he also had a new startup brewing. As predicted, the two men got into an animated conversation. But they were on parallel tracks that never intersected. John talked about the Words Project, and Frank talked about spinal manipulation. Just as one Gorman paused for breath, the other would jump in and continue what he was saying. Julia had heard similar discussions among other Gorman men, recalling Kevin Gorman's focus on gravity. "The Gormans are a fixated bunch," Julia said to Kath. "Ah yes, they're a bright lot," Kath nodded, spiriting Julia away for tea.

John had only fond memories of Sydney, starting off when he and classmate John Hamilton hitchhiked into town. The Eleventh Congress of the International Society of Blood Transfusion of 1966 had been unforgettable, with the announcements of the imminent breakthrough in Rh disease. And he had spent time at the blood bank in Sydney as well as in several centers across Australia, advising doctors and staff on how to get the most out of their Rh programs. He would never forget how quickly the country had recruited donors, created anti-D, and made it available to women in need. In one letter to Dr. Gordon Archer at the Sydney blood bank, Gorman wrote: "Usage figures in Australia are better than anywhere else in the world."

Toward the end of his Australia visit, John, a diligent reader of newspapers, came across a story about the success of the Rh program in Australia. The story told some of the history and spotlighted a "super donor" named James Harrison, who had become known as "the Man with the Golden Arm." John read about how this man received an Australian medal of honor and was in the *Guinness World Records* book for his blood donations. In the story, Harrison was quoted as saying, "I'm not a hero. All I do is sit back in a chair and stick out my arm." The story ended by asking for "future heroes" to step forward and donate blood.

John had heard of James Harrison, and he'd spent a good amount of time with Dr. Archer and the team from the Sydney blood bank, where Harrison made most of his donations. At one point, John remembered being shown the records of the Sydney donors. The records consisted of note cards with handwritten entries, like the ones he had created at Sing Sing to track names, blood types, injection dates, and antibody responses. He remembered Archer talking in those early days about Harrison as an unusual donor. His impressive antibodies were said to be the result of a lifesaving surgery he had as a teenager. It made perfect sense to John: As a youth, James Harrison was washed with Rh-positive blood.

Decades after that surgery, when James Harrison was injected again with Rh-positive blood as a part of the Rh program, his antibodies jumped back into action. John said he had seen the same thing happen, to a lesser degree, with the men at Sing Sing. Two years after the prisoners were last boosted, one small injection of red blood cells would prompt their antibody levels to jump up again. As John had explained to the prisoners at the time: "The antibody factory goes to sleep for lack of stimulus, but it jumps back up when faced with the same antigen." This was *immunological memory*, where the immune system remembers antigens that previously activated a response. With subsequent exposures to the same antigen, increasingly intense responses were activated. The more the body recognized the invader, the swifter and more lethal its response.

John had told Dr. Archer and the team at the Sydney blood center: "Some people you can't immunize. You give them multiple shots and no antibodies. Others make enormous titers." John recalled looking over James Harrison's donor cards and thinking, "Here is a donor who is making a lot of antibodies. If a mother had those levels, her baby would never survive."

But what John found most impressive, even back then, was that this donor, James Harrison, never missed a donation. John told Dr.

Archer: "This is what we call a superb source." And he marveled, "He must have a lot of stamina."

John thought about what it meant to have a donor like James Harrison. John had spent decades in blood banks and had never come across anyone like this. His office at Columbia had been in the donor room, which is where he'd first spotted Carol. It's where he'd met the irrepressible Vince Freda. It's where he'd started out on this Rh journey. But it was also where he saw the day-to-day workings of blood banks: of nurses or medical students sometimes struggling to find a vein, of being called in himself to find the vein, of grumpy donors, unpredictable donors, rescheduled appointments, and donors who fainted from the loss of blood—something that happened with great frequency, as donors weren't getting enough blood to the brain. John would try to explain that a blood draw was the same as bleeding out—the only difference was this was into a bag.

It dawned on John now, sitting with sister-in-law Kath in her kitchen and surrounded by photos of their kids and grandkids, that it would have been James Harrison's blood that had saved the lives of Kath and Frank's three older children, Friedel, Giles, and Jacob. They were all born in Australia. They would all have been protected by James Harrison's antibodies. The man had been donating for six decades. *Now here is a hero*, John thought.

On the flight home to California, John thought again about James Harrison, and he reflected on the heroic acts of his own family—his mother, father, some of his forebears, and many of his relatives. Vince Freda, who had passed away, had dedicated his life to ending Rh disease. He was a hero. James Harrison, "the Man with the Golden Arm," was absolutely a hero. Harrison's defiant stand was simply showing up for something he believed in. Again and again. Year after year. Decade after decade. But he was brave, too, enduring discomfort and some level of risk to help others. He was, John realized, that noble character with special powers. His blood was lifesaving, his determination life affirming.

John's journey had always been more about the intellect, from the very beginning. Move the figurine on the tray of the highchair and win dad's approval. Memorize mathematical equations, names of cities, capitals, countries. Turn vacuum tubes into radios, a piece of wood into a boomerang. Build a better prothrombin test. Better blood-banking software. More sentient computers. Find an answer to a dangerous riddle of the immune system.

John Gorman had been pulled into Rh through his mind. James Harrison had been drawn in because of his heart. Though the two men had never met—and lived continents apart—they had worked together for a higher purpose. Maybe together, John thought, they had achieved something heroic.

John pulled down the window shade to get some rest. His mind returned to the day he left Melbourne to chase his dreams in America, to the moment when the white streamer held by his mother broke and he was on his own. The thin and ethereal bands floated around him.

His parents, and their acts of heroism, had shaped him in ways that he'd never fathomed before. It had been sixty years since he had sailed for America, but his voyage of discovery hadn't ended. He was still learning about science. About humanity. About inventions that could make a difference. And most important, about himself.

CHAPTER TWENTY-THREE
The Infinite Lifeline

James Harrison watched the changing landscape through the train window. From time to time, he could spot kids playing cricket in a schoolyard. Catching his reflection in the glass, James still felt like the same rascal in Junee forever angling to get outside to play with his mates. But his hair was now gray, and he was dressed in brown trousers, a short-sleeve white shirt, and a brown-and-white striped tie. He was on his way from his home in Umina Beach to the blood bank in Sydney, a route he'd taken hundreds of times. But this day was unlike any other.

In the hills across the sparkling Sydney Harbour and bridge, Robyn Barlow spent a bit of extra time getting ready, doing her hair and makeup and choosing her wardrobe carefully. She set a small box by the door. Inside was a treasure she didn't want to forget.

Not faraway, in suburban Waverton, retired nurse Lizzie Thynne talked to her canaries before heading out the door of her apartment and down to the street, where she would catch a ride to the Sydney blood center. She had developed vertigo and hadn't been out much lately. But she was not about to miss today.

James's train ride to Sydney from Woy Woy, the station closest to Umina Beach, took about ninety minutes. The route was as familiar to James as his oldest stamps, taking him through gorgeous mountain terrain and across the Hawkesbury River before slicing through several national parks. There were stops along the way, with the rush of commuters on and off platforms, and sleepy towns reminiscent of the 1950s.

Arriving at the Town Hall station under George Street, where the Sydney blood center was now located, James climbed the stairs to the street. It was a gorgeous day, and the sunlight reflected off the impressive buildings, including the ornate nineteenth-century Town Hall offices, home to the mayor and city officials. James slowed to a stop as he neared the entrance to the blood bank. Television trucks were parked along the front of the building. He could see a crowd had gathered inside.

It was May 11, 2018, and James wished it were just a normal day of donating. Walking into the blood center, he was buoyed by the familiar faces: Robyn; Lizzie; his daughter, Tracey, and son-in-law, Andrew; and the blood center staff. Television cameras began recording James's every move: as he said his hellos, signed in, had his blood pressure taken, took a seat in a reclining brown chair, and was handed a red foam heart to squeeze in his right hand.

Except for the cameras trained on him, this was all familiar territory: the attentive nurses, nearby donors, gauze bandages, alcohol prep pads, needles, rubber gloves. The plasmapheresis machine was moved to James's right. The nurse palpated James's arm and used an alcohol prep pad, swabbing the intended injection site from the center to periphery. The nurse held the needle at a thirty-degree angle to the surface of James's arm, and then slid it through the skin and into the vein. The crook of James's arm was the best bullseye around.

Never one to watch the needle enter his skin, James had plenty to distract himself with today. "One thing that will never change," he said, "is I can't stand the sight of blood." This was quite a statement, considering the magnitude of the day.

James Christopher Harrison was making his 1,173rd blood donation. It would be his last. He was eighty-one years old and had reached the cutoff age for donating blood in Australia.

One by one, as James had his blood drawn, a dozen mothers and a handful of fathers holding their babies approached to thank him. A baby girl reached out to feel James's whiskers. A baby boy in a blue knit cap giggled when James made a funny face. Another baby appeared to have his sights set on the glasses in James's left shirt pocket. Behind James were four big Mylar balloons forming the number 1173. All but 10 of the 1,173 donations had come from James's right arm.

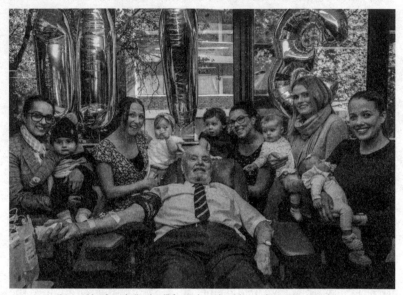

James Harrison is "retired" from donating blood after 1,173 donations.

As the dark red blood left James's body, the plasmapheresis machine separated the blood into one bag of honey-colored plasma and another bag of red cells that would be returned to him. James chatted easily with the moms and dads gathered for the occasion. A gallery of people watched and took photos. Tracey was content to stay at the back of the room. It was her dad's day.

A young mother told James: "Early in my pregnancy, I was told I needed the vaccine. I didn't know much about Rh. Then I learned about you."

A dad standing nearby said, "If it weren't for you, James, our baby girl wouldn't be here."

James replied, "I guess you can blame me for Australia's over-population!"

Another mom, who had anti-D injections during her second pregnancy, said, "You are remarkable. We don't even hear of Rh disease today because the treatment is so effective."

The parents gathered in the Town Hall Blood Centre represented a drop of water in the sea of lives saved by James's unique, disease-fighting antibodies. Most of the young parents didn't know much about Rh disease because they didn't need to; it wasn't a problem anymore. As a part of their prenatal care, expectant mothers with an Rh incompatibility were told by their doctors that they would need two anti-D injections—one during pregnancy and one within seventy-two hours of delivery. But there was nothing to worry about. The treatment was entirely safe and effective.

The mothers and fathers in the room knew little of the problems and grief they may have faced without anti-D, or what life looked like to Rh-incompatible mothers and fathers who had babies before the treatment was available. They could not have known of the incremental steps forward over decades in the understanding of blood, blood typing, transfusions, immunology, prenatal care, and Rh disease. They would not have known of the eureka moment when a young Australian doctor, working in a blood bank in New York City, read a paragraph in a textbook and landed on a contrarian idea about using passive antibodies to stop Rh, or of how that idea was dismissed long before it was embraced.

There were hundreds of small victories that led to this day. There were the Rh blood trials involving prisoners in Sing Sing, and the first trials in England involving policemen who volunteered to be human guinea pigs. There were the mothers who had endured horrific losses from Rh but emerged from their despair to try to prevent other mothers from suffering the same fate. The parents filling the blood center would not have known that the seventy-two-hour protocol for the second injection was decided by a warden at Sing Sing concerned with prison breakouts, not by clinical studies or deep medical reasoning. And no one would have imagined that James Harrison's blood was ever deemed *subpar* and unsuitable for human transfusions. Only later—after the eureka moment by researcher and pathologist John Gorman in New York— was it discovered that James's blood was rich in the supercharged antibodies needed to combat Rh.

"James thinks his donations are the same as anybody else," a director of the blood center said, standing next to James. "But he's a national hero."

James demurred, saying, "No, no, no. It's just something I can do. It's one of my talents. Probably my only talent."

James remembered one of his very first donations—more than six decades earlier—when a nurse told him he had "the loveliest veins." When he was even younger, a nurse at St. Vincent's Hospital told him in the days before his surgery, when he was weak and ill, that his veins were as "strong as the Australian sun in summertime." Under his shirt was the winding scar that snaked from his sternum to the middle of his back. Etched into his skin by more than one hundred stitches following his surgery, the scar was now a thin and faded line.

Another mom at the blood center approached James and gave him a card that she and her kids had made. It read: "Heroes don't wear capes. Heroes donate blood and save lives." James said it was lovely. A dad shook James's left hand and told him he deserved "the Nobel Prize for generosity."

Robyn, who had been off to the side visiting with nurse Lizzie, saw her opportunity and made her way through the TV cameras and well-wishers. Reaching James, whose blood was still being drawn, she wrapped her arms around his shoulders and hugged him tightly.

"It's sort of sad," she said, unexpectedly breaking into tears.

"It is sad, yes," James said, holding on to her.

"We were here at the beginning," Robyn said, standing back and wiping away the tears. "We're here at the end, who would think?"

Turning to the parents, Robyn said, "Every ampule of anti-D ever made in Australia has James in it. I cry just thinking about it."

She then looked at the comfy recliner and joked with James, "No feet out the window here."

Robyn searched in her purse for the white box she'd brought from home. The treasure inside was James's donation cards, relics connecting past to present. The 5x7 cards in pale green, pink, and light blue were worn at the edges with handwritten notes and the occasional coffee stain. They dated to the beginning of the Rh program in Australia in 1967, following the announcements a year earlier of the breakthrough research and trials in Rh disease at the Eleventh Congress of the International Society of Blood Transfusion. The first donation card had basic information: "James Christopher Harrison, blood type O negative, Pre-Immunized." Toward the bottom of the card, written

James Harrison's blood donation cards from the early days of the Rh program in Australia.

in pencil in cursive, was "lobectomy 1951," referring to James's lung surgery at age fourteen, when massive transfusions saved his life and supercharged his blood.

In the blood center, as the TV cameras rolled, the bag containing James's plasma filled up and was taken away. The blood would be sent to the lab for freezing at –20 degrees Celsius (–4°F), then transported to Melbourne to be processed into the anti-D treatment and shipped across Australia. Roughly 17 percent of pregnant women in Australia received anti-D. It remained the only preventative treatment for Rh disease, and the only source was donors with anti-Rh antibodies.

Robyn kept all of James's news clippings as well as the records and dates of his milestones as an Rh donor: 100 donations as of June 1973; 200 donations as of May 1979; 300 donations as of May 1983; 400 donations as of August 1987; 500 donations as of June 1991; 600 donations as of June 1995; 700 donations as of April 1999; 800 donations as of January 2003; 900 donations as of February 2007; and 1,000 donations as of May 2011, when grandson Scott joined him.

Now a staggering new tally had been generated by the Australian Red Cross. The number was 2.4 million. Through his 1,173 donations over sixty-two years, James had saved the lives of more than 2.4 million babies.

One man. Two million four hundred thousand lives saved. What had started at age eighteen was ending at age eighty-one.

The last donation was made. James held the cotton swab down, and the nurse applied the gauze bandage. Moms and dads continued to come by to thank him. Several asked whether he would hold their babies. He held up a smiling baby girl. He cradled twins, one in each arm. He held a big baby boy, born eleven pounds, five ounces, his proud mother said. But soon the cameras were turned off and the television trucks began pulling away. James paused for more photos in the blood center café, which had been named after him—with a plaque reading

"The James Harrison Café, Australia's Greatest Donor, 1173 Blood Donations"—before heading to lunch with Tracey, Andrew, Robyn, Lizzie, and a small team from the blood bank.

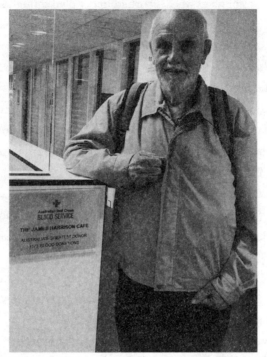

James Harrison in the summer of 2019, visiting the blood donation center in Sydney, where the café has been named after him.

James walked beside Tracey, lost in thought. Two million-plus babies was a hard number to grasp. The number included his own grandson and his sister Margaret's children. James wondered: *How many people are lucky enough to save one life?* Donating a kidney to a stranger was amazing. Plucking someone from a burning building took split-second processing and bravery. But James had no frame of reference for 2.4 million lives *saved*. History was rife with stories of vast numbers of lives *taken* by despots and in genocides, whether during the Holocaust or in Cambodia, Rwanda, Darfur, Bosnia, and many other places. *But what protected life?* Beyond medical breakthroughs, technological advancements, contrarian ideas, and knowledge, James had his own answer: kindness.

Tracey was quiet as well, absorbed in her own thoughts. She knew how proud her mom would have been that day. Barb would have stayed at the back of the room with her, happy to let her "gorgeous man" shine. Tracey hadn't told her dad this yet, but she had started having dreams in which she saw her mom. The dreams were always the same: Tracey was stressed about something, but when her mom appeared, Tracey knew everything would be okay. In some dreams, her mom and dad were together, and Tracey was comforted in the same way. She had never had dreams like this before.

"We had a good run," James said finally, pulled from his miasma as they walked from the blood center on George Street to the ArtHouse Hotel on Pitt Street. The Red Cross was treating James and friends to lunch.

"Yes, it feels like the end of an era," Robyn said. "But what an era—2.4 million babies! Not many people can say that, now can they?"

"Not bad for a country lad," James nodded.

It had been fifty years since RhoGAM was approved in the United States and Australia began producing anti-D. Globally, tens of millions of lives had been saved by the anti-Rh injections. The number of lives saved would continue to grow for as long as the disease exists. With the elimination of these once high-risk pregnancies, billions of dollars were saved, and there have been no fatalities linked to the anti-Rh treatments.

Taking his seat in the restaurant, James told Lizzie that it felt like forever since they'd last seen each other. She had retired in 2013, five years earlier, at age seventy.

"I didn't want to leave, either," Lizzie said. "I had worked all my life, since I was seventeen. Toward the end, people kept saying to me,

'You're not tired, are you?' I wasn't tired at all! But they gave me a terrific farewell. Everyone brought flowers. I was there for most of a half century."

"I had said I wouldn't stop until the well ran dry," James said. "Or until they had to use two hands to get the needle into the vein. But neither happened. I would've kept going. But once you turn eighty-one, they determine your blood's not worth bottling."

Lizzie nodded. "It's a sad day alright. Sad that there's a knockoff age of eighty-one. But you do have to look after the person, too."

"Time moves on," Robyn said.

"I was so attached to all the donors," Lizzie lamented. "I had donors say to me, 'Liz, you make me laugh.'"

Lizzie had always worked hard to make the blood center feel welcoming. She spent her own money on flowers for the reception area. She was known to dash out of the center to help donors with taxi fare—again out of her own pocket. She gave some of her baby chicks to donors who expressed interest, and attended birthday parties, funerals, and holiday events with donors. She was invited to Olive Semmler's seventieth birthday party in. "She made the best sponge cake with cream and jelly and who knows what," Lizzie said dreamily.

"Olive was a strong woman," James said. "A good lady. An inspiration."

"She was gorgeous," Lizzie said. "Gorgeous in love with her husband—a big tall farmer. A quiet man. They had been through so much together. It was sad when he died. Cancer. He lived a healthy life, never smoked or drank. Their daughter, Val, had wondered whether her dad's stress of worrying about Olive and the babies and never having anyone to share his feelings with contributed to the cancer."

James remembered when he first met Lizzie and took to calling her a "sticky beak." She was as cheerful, chatty, and guileless today as back in the day.

"Olive told me that she almost died with the seventh pregnancy," Lizzie continued. "She was rushed by helicopter to Sydney and was very ill. She lost the baby. Only her mom, daughter, Val, and husband could see her. She was moved to this wing where she was by herself and said she would have died had it not been for one nurse who sat with her, made her eat, and brought her back to life."

"She was proud she made it to five hundred donations," Robyn said. "She always kept her five hundred-donations badge with her."

"They all have good souls," Lizzie said of the donors.

"They believe in doing the right thing," said Robyn.

"And they're good looking," James added, making everyone laugh.

Lizzie took the bait, saying, "James was very handsome. Dark hair. Very good looking."

James protested: "*Was* very handsome?"

Lizzie and Robyn shared stories about more of the regulars. There was the "bag lady," who brought in the purses she'd made to sell, and the "frog lady," who was married to a scientist who studied frogs. Then there was the woman donor who was blind. Her husband brought her in regularly to donate. "She said her life was blessed and she wanted to give back," Lizzie marveled. Another regular donor was a caregiver for her elderly husband. Coming in to donate blood was a welcome break for her. "She and I would sit and chat away," Lizzie said, happy in the memories.

Robyn, who had been mostly quiet, said, "What we did here you could never do again."

The bold statement got everyone's attention at the lunch table. "For starters," Robyn continued, "to have one donor, our very own James Harrison, remain well and fit and have veins strong enough to continue to donate for so long is very, very rare."

James nodded. "Thank you, Robyn."

"But also, Rh broke *all the rules*," she said. "John Gorman and Vince Freda, the brilliant researchers in New York certainly broke the rules by sending their experimental ampule from America to England, without approval from anyone. Their tests on the prisoners at Sing Sing were crucial for this whole thing. But those trials would never be allowed to happen now. And what the English researchers did with the policemen who volunteered was the same. You had researchers injecting themselves with the Rh-positive blood first, to show the volunteers it was safe. Then you had these men who took big risks, not knowing how their own bodies would react to the injections. Again, this would never happen now."

Robyn first met John Gorman when he visited the Sydney blood bank at 1 York Street to work with her boss, Gordon Archer, and to offer expertise on setting up the Rh program.

"Ah, yes, he's the Aussie from Bendigo, right?" James asked.

"Yes, and he's just brilliant—and very humble," Robyn said, explaining that she and Dr. Archer had lunch with Gorman in New York in the mid-eighties, when the two men were speaking at a conference. Over lunch, she heard stories about Vince Freda, Sing Sing, Kath, and more.

Robyn remembered the time when Gorman visited the Sydney blood center, instructing everyone to find women donors who had the anti-D antibodies. Looking right at James, Robyn said: "Then he told us we should find male donors who were Rh negative. Gorman explained how we could boost their blood, at what intervals, and all that was needed."

"That's when they found *me*," James said proudly. "I thought maybe I was in trouble when they called me in. But I was being named the star student."

Robyn rolled her eyes and smiled. She and James had become like brother and sister.

"We never had to have a clinical trial of our own," Robyn continued, "because it had already been done. The man who did it was our adviser! There were all these things you just wouldn't be able to do today. Plus, in those days, no one would think of suing anyone."

Robyn, growing emotional again, said that when passing by a schoolyard or a playground, she sometimes imagined taking away the kids who would not have been there had it not been for James. "I can tell you one thing with confidence," she said. "We'll never see the likes of James again."

James found himself blushing. The only thing missing from this day was Barb. She had always implored him to be kind—and he would never have been able to complete his sixty-year donor journey without her. As Robyn continued to gush about him, he felt even more humbled.

"Saved lives can become common, medicine taken for granted, like what happened with penicillin or polio or TB," Robyn said. "Sure, James looks like an ordinary guy. Most people have never heard of him. He doesn't wear a cape. He doesn't have a shield. What does he have? He has a bandage on his arm. Under the bandage is scar tissue from where he's donated blood for sixty years."

Looking at James, Lizzie, Tracey, and the others, Robyn raised her glass and said, "Everything that was right and true happened here."

Lizzie nodded. "I always felt that I was doing something important," she said. "Through all the tragedy, if you can look after people who've been hurting, it's wonderful. I feel like I was meant to be there."

Robyn, too, believed she had been somehow steered to the blood center. She had no prior experience as a nurse or in any medical capacity, but she could not have been better suited for the job. She held on to her belief that the breakthrough with Rh was one of the greatest lifesaving discoveries of the twentieth century.

James listened with interest. He had never been one to stop and analyze or spend much time in reflection, always abiding by the Hank

Williams saying: "If a song can't be written in twenty minutes, it ain't worth writing." But he was moved by the words of his friends and the outpouring of gratitude from strangers.

The lunch celebration passed too quickly. Plates were removed, coffee cups drained. Everyone began packing up their things. Lizzie would get a ride home from a friend. Tracey was headed back to work. Robyn had her car but would walk with James to the railway station. On the street, everyone said their goodbyes, knowing they would always be connected by Rh.

Back at the Town Hall station on George Street, Robyn and James embraced one more time. Then Robyn headed off, turning once to look back and smile and wave. James watched her walk away. *She's a lovely girl.* He made his way through the busy square. Just before heading down the stairs, he heard "Mr. Harrison! Mr. Harrison!" It was one of the moms who had been at the event and was hurrying toward him, pushing her twins in the stroller. She asked whether she could give him another hug.

"Of course," James said. The two had a warm exchange before James made his way down to the platform.

Finally, back on the train, James exhaled. *What a day!* He was tired, energized, proud, grateful, overwhelmed, melancholy, and happy all at once.

The stories played in his mind. Lizzie said her losses—the loss of her own mother and the grief that followed—had made her *better at giving, better at loving.* James believed that Olive Semmler was the same. Olive had turned something terrible that took baby after baby from her and made something positive. Robyn said she had found her calling in the blood bank, energized by a lifesaving mission. She was changed by the resilience of the women donors who could not lift their gaze off the floor when she first met them but would later march in with heads held high, determined to help. And as Robyn said, James had to nearly lose his life to be able to give life to others. What had started for him as a duty ended as a privilege.

Feeling the tender crook of his arm where the needle had been, James knew that the day would come when his blood would stop pumping. But just as he had been given a second chance at life, there were now millions of babies protected by his antibodies. Many would go on to have their own children, and those children in turn would have children, too. The 2.4 million would multiply, and the lifeline was infinite. James relaxed into his seat. He smiled thinking of what he had told the mother of the twins.

"There's a little bit of me in your babies," James said, "so look after them for me."

EPILOGUE
A War Still Being Waged

"Wasn't Rh disease cured fifty years ago?"

That's a question I recently got from a doctor friend upon hearing the subject of this book.

"Well, yes—and no," I said. "There is no cure, but there is a treatment that is nearly 100 percent effective."

Then I had to add: "But not all women are getting the injections they need to protect their babies."

In fact, consider this: Globally, only 50 percent of women at risk for Rh disease each year are receiving the anti-Rh injections they need. With an estimated 5 million pregnancies at risk for Rh disease each year, this means that some 2.5 million women are not receiving any treatment at all.

"We have a drug that works perfectly, with no side effects," said Steven Spitalnik, a director of the laboratory of transfusion biology and professor of pathology and cell biology at Columbia University Medical Center. "But it is not getting to women in developing countries."

In the most modernized nations, pregnant women routinely get an Rh blood test as part of their prenatal care and then routinely receive an anti-D injection during pregnancy and another following birth. Because of this standard procedure, Rh disease has virtually disappeared from Western Europe, Canada, the United States, and Australia.

But in developing countries, Rh disease is still common due to the lack of access to high-quality health care—and perhaps even more alarmingly, a lack of awareness of the problem and the solution. The breakthrough treatment, available for more than a half a century, is not getting to Rh-negative women in most African countries, China, Pakistan, parts of South America, and more. These nations represent more than 40 percent of the world's population.

The problem is, Rh can only be screened for if mothers know their blood type and know the father's blood type. The disease can only be reported to health officials and tallied by world health organizations if diagnosed, another challenge in countries where babies die unreported and autopsies are seldom if ever performed. And the signs of Rh disease—stillbirths, anemia, jaundice, swelling under the skin—can be attributed to many possible causes.

"Even though I'm a blood banker and we give our Rh immunoglobulin regularly, I've seen few cases of Rh in my career," said Spitalnik, the pathology professor at Columbia. "The cases I have seen in New York were in the immigrant community, with mothers from the Dominican Republic. But I thought this disease was done. It didn't strike me as a major problem."

Spitalnik said he had an "awakening" to the ongoing problems of Rh in early 2018 when he was organizing the fifty-year anniversary events around the approval of RhoGAM in the United States. The celebration at Columbia involved John Gorman, Vince Freda's family, Marianne Cummins and her husband, Dennis, family members of the Liverpool scientists, and others who were involved in research, trials, and discovery of the Rh treatment.

"I had my consciousness raised to the reality that although it may have been solved in the United States, it hasn't been solved in the rest of the world," Spitalnik said.

He added, "This results in a continuing burden of fetal and neonatal disease, and tremendous emotional distress to far too many women and their families across the globe, particularly in South and Central America, Africa, and Southeast Asia. It is even more distressing that some women and children in the high-income countries of

Europe and North America are still affected by this completely pre-ventable disease."

Canadian researcher Alvin Zipursky, who was at the vanguard of Canada's effort to combat Rh and is often called a "rock star" of hematology, had a similar awakening years earlier to the persistent problems of Rh. He is eighty-nine but says he will not be able to fully retire until Rh disease is vanquished across the globe. "It's a real scourge, and it's solvable," Zipursky says. "My goal is very modest. Wipe out Rh disease worldwide."

Through his connections with doctors in Canada, Stanford University in California, and Columbia in New York, Zipursky helped launch an early consortium with pilot projects in Ghana and India. At one Ghanaian hospital alone, about two hundred babies a year are affected by Rh disease.

More recently, Spitalnik helped found the Worldwide Initiative for Rh Disease Eradication (WIRhE), an international group of physicians, scientists, midwives, global health advocates, and corporate partners committed to ridding the globe of Rh disease. Spitalnik serves as executive director, and the group has studies and early programs taking shape in China, Russia, Pakistan, and Nigeria.

But the challenges are deep-rooted and different for each country, from trying to educate midwives in remote areas of Russia to getting safe access to clinics and doctors in Pakistan. Spitalnik points out: "If you are the minister of health in the Congo and I tell you that none of the Rh-negative women in your country are being protected and you have that burden of disease, you may come back to me and say, 'Yes, and I have AIDS and Ebola and war and malaria.' Hearing that, I know that those are real issues. So, we have learned that we need to make it so easy and low cost that there is no burden to implementing."

In Nigeria, another area of study—Rhesus disease is lower among Africans than Caucasians—there are an estimated thirty-three thousand cases of Rh disease per year. For this African nation, the underlying challenges of providing access to anti-Rh are poverty and awareness. More than half the women who deliver babies in Nigeria do not see a health care provider before giving birth. Even the women who know they need the injection can't afford it. Many women flee from hospitals or health clinics with their babies out of fear of the costs. The obstetrical horror stories coming from women in Nigeria remind Zipursky of stories he heard decades earlier from his "Rh Ladies of Winnipeg" in Canada. The location is different, but the loss feels the same.

Zipursky tells the story of Florence Onwuasoanya in Nigeria, who became known in her community as "the woman who loses all the babies." She lost nine babies—some arrived stillborn, others were miscarriages. Her husband responded by taking another wife. Florence was made to think she was cursed. She sought out exorcism rituals and tried a range of concoctions that did nothing but make her sick. Then one day, visiting a new clinic, she learned about Rh disease. She has become an advocate for Rh awareness, saying, "I don't want any woman to go through what I went through."

Spitalnik and Zipursky and the group from WIRhE are working to raise money and awareness around the battle against Rh—a war they thought was already won.

"We're writing papers, translating our work into Spanish and Russian and other languages, and finding ways into Pakistan and China and elsewhere," Spitalnik said. "But in the meantime, we're setting our sights on protecting ten thousand women this year who otherwise would not be protected. It's not 2.5 million, but it's a start."

JOHN GORMAN WAS RECENTLY in New York for a Lasker Awards luncheon. Afterward, he took the subway to head to Columbia for meetings with Steve Spitalnik and others. He realized he had plenty of time before the meetings to revisit an old haunt, so got out of the subway at Columbus Circle and walked over to the fabled Oak Room for a martini.

Arriving at the Plaza Hotel, he was dismayed to find that the Oak Room had been closed—again—for another round of renovations. Heading back out onto the street, he decided to go across to the Four Seasons at Fifty-Seventh Street.

Taking a seat at the gorgeous Four Seasons bar, he ordered a martini. The bill arrived, and John had to look twice to make sure he was reading correctly. The martini was $32.

John said to the guy sitting next to him: "I used to get a martini for $1.25!"

The guy nodded and said, "It's very expensive to get drunk in New York."

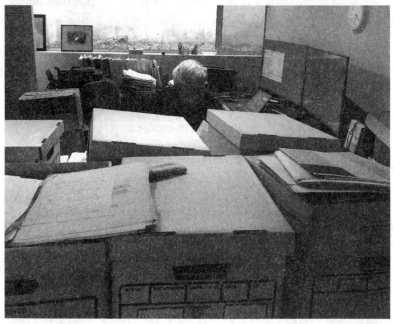

John Gorman at his home near San Diego, California, surrounded by boxes filled with his Rh research. The papers will soon go into the archives of Columbia University.

John laughed, nodding in appreciation. The hefty bill reminded him of why he had decided to leave the hustle and bustle of Manhattan decades earlier, though he would always have a soft spot for the place where he found his great loves, raised his wonderful children—and made a profound difference in fighting a scourge that has plagued the world.

Even being far away from New York, as a purportedly retired transplant in California, John has not slowed down in his quest to make better blood for humankind.

These days, at age eighty-nine, he is energized by his newest invention to improve blood banking. He has incorporated a startup called Team Conveyor Intellectual Properties, with two technology patents pending.

"I've always wanted to improve the automation of blood bank testing," he said over lunch, back home in Del Mar, California, not far from San Diego. "The work I've done around this before wasn't the right approach. Since then, I've thought of a much better way to do automation. It's very different from anything that exists. It's good for blood banks and good for all clinical lab tests. It will be ten times better and one hundred times faster."

John had barely sat down for lunch before he began arranging the salt and pepper shakers and other jars and containers on a carousel in front of him. "All robotics are on a pull system," he said, moving the carousel, clearly lost in his idea. "My idea is a push system."

His wife, Julia, could only smile. The gleam in his eyes was familiar: a new obsession had taken hold. When he wasn't tinkering on the startup, John and Julia continued to enjoy their life together. They take walks on the beach and savor their routines of tea in the morning, lunch at noon, and one martini in the early evening. They are working on their golf games, and visit regularly with their kids and six grandkids. Daughter Elizabeth Gorman works for Federated Investors in New York.

Son John "Cito" Gorman is director of the SolarNetwork Foundation in New Zealand. Daughter Alex Scranton is the director of science and research at Women's Voices for the Earth in Montana. And stepson Lorenzo Cavalletti runs an internet sales business. Family photos are prominent throughout the Del Mar house.

But even as John could opt for more leisure time, his mind today is clearly on this latest invention. He talks about the size of the blood bank industry—"It's enormous, $330 billion in 2026"—and the critical need to improve efficiency in the testing of blood. It's an invention that could have ramifications for identifying and fighting diseases worldwide, including Rh.

"Blood banking is behind in the technology by around forty years," he says. "They're starting to automate, but I've come up with a much better way." Then he launches into his unorthodox thinking around raising capital for the startup, saying, "I've decided we're going to have a million units and that's all there ever will be. And you can only get shares by buying them from founders."

John hurries through his lunch so that he can return to his startup. "The company is an idea company," he says. "The best ideas are simple, hanging out there like fruit. You just have to be able to see them." Inventing is often about reimagining something that already exists. The Band-Aid started by putting together gauze and surgical tape. The Slinky was born out of a bundle of wires. Vacutainers were tubes with a colored rubber stopper and vacuum seal. Ketchup existed for decades before someone thought to turn the bottle upside down. The gas cap tank became so much better when a simple tether was attached.

Yet this man of ideas has never forgotten the most important, uncannily simple idea that he ever had: that passive Rh antibodies could combat the disease and save millions of babies. Signs of his incredible journey of discovery abound in the Del Mar house. The shelves in the downstairs office are filled with boxes of archival materials from his days at Columbia and his years doing Rh research and trials. He has stacks of letters from mothers who wrote to him after hearing that a breakthrough treatment for Rh disease was imminent. He has handwritten records from the Sing Sing trials, notes from and to Vince Freda and Bill Pollack, and piles of research papers and related articles. Columbia University, which recently established the Gorman Lecture Series, has asked for John's archives for its permanent collection.

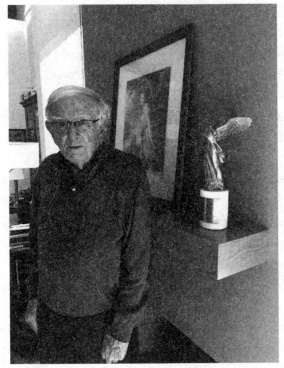

John Gorman at home in late 2019, with the Lasker Award trophy on the fireplace mantel.

On John's fireplace mantel, in the upstairs living room, is the Lasker Award trophy, won in 1980 by John, Vince, Bill Pollack, and the team from Liverpool. Never far from John is the copy of the book *Ideas*

Have Consequences, which he brought with him when he boarded the ship from Melbourne to America. The book was a gift from his father.

As he says now, "I'm absolutely thrilled when a good idea takes off. I do love ideas with consequences."

JAMES HARRISON CONTINUES TO have his celebrity moments in Australia. He was recently invited to morning tea with the governor of New South Wales—part of an honor in which he was named one of the country's best senior citizens of the year.

As James enjoyed tea and biscuits at the governor's mansion in Sydney, the Honorable Margaret Beazley talked to James about Rh. She asked him questions about his blood donations over the years and then talked about her own career—she was known to be a role model for women in law. She also talked about her three children, Erin, Lauren, and Anthony Sullivan. She surprised James by saying, "I had your anti-D injections for my three children."

"Then we're almost related!" James declared.

James also recently got a call from researchers at the blood bank in Sydney who asked to send someone to collect more of his blood. Australian scientists are working on a program called "James in a Jar," to try to create a synthetic anti-D antibody mimicking the antibodies found in James's blood.

Efforts have been underway for several years, but to date, no amount of genetic engineering has been able to match the antibodies in James's blood. And more than a half-century after the treatment was approved for use, no one knows exactly how antibodies like James's work to protect the mother.

"I never know where I am going to be when someone says they've got my anti-D," James tells his friends. "I am still getting this from people all the time."

On a Sunday in mid-January 2020, James spends his morning

preparing lunch at his home in Umina Beach. He has just come back from the store, where he has purchased ham, cheese, eggs, tomatoes, and lettuce. A special guest is coming over.

When everything is ready—as if on cue—in walks Joy Maidment, who lives just up the road.

James and Joy met years earlier at a Probus Club luncheon held in their neighborhood. James and Joy got to chatting during the lunch, and James learned that Joy had lost her husband around the same time he lost Barb. It turned out that they live close to one another and have many shared interests, including stamp collecting. Joy talked with pride about her two grown children and two grandchildren.

After the Probus Club luncheon, James decided to invite Joy to a stamp meeting. He again found her easy to talk to and enjoyed her company.

James now calls Joy his "best friend."

"Joy turns eighty this spring," he says, "so I'm not snatching anyone from a cradle." And with a wink, he adds, "We told our respective children we wouldn't be having children, so their inheritance is quite safe."

James and Joy keep their separate houses but call to check on each other every morning. James, always ready with a joke about almost anything, including getting older, quips: "I don't buy any green bananas." And when he greets people his age, he likes to say, "You look well for a person your age." He still doesn't know how to cook, though he has become something of an expert at boiling water and defrosting vegetables in the microwave.

"I have a George Foreman grill, so I can cook a steak," he says proudly.

He and Joy keep busy with their clubs and hobbies and trade off treating one another to lunch at home, just like they are doing today. Like everyone else, Joy was impressed to learn of James's history as a blood donor. But James, whose dedication and superhuman blood saved millions of babies, continues to handle such compliments with his trademark understatement and self-deprecating humor. It's the only way he knows how.

"She thought what I had done was pretty good," he says of his donating. "She had something to tell her grandkids about."

AUTHOR'S NOTE

My path to this new book, *Good Blood*, began when I read a short item in the *New York Times* about "the Man with the Golden Arm" being retired after donating blood for more than sixty years, saving 2.4 million babies in his native Australia. The news item caught my attention because of my interest in how ordinary people do extraordinary things.

The more I delved into the story, the more I became captivated by this bookkeeper for the railroad who had somehow saved millions of lives with his "special blood." I wanted to know more: How did James Harrison become such a hero in this lifesaving endeavor? How did the world of science find James? What is Rh disease, and as a mother and journalist who chronicled people of science and health, why had I never heard of it? How can *one person* possibly save 2.4 million babies?

I tracked James Harrison down through the Red Cross Donor Service in Sydney, Australia, and was charmed and inspired from our first phone call. I found him funny, wise, and humble. Our conversations were filled with his Aussie aphorisms that I find especially refreshing today. James's story felt so resonant because he reminds us of what is important in life. He was never after money or fame. He never accepted a penny for his valuable blood. He wouldn't know how to tweet, post, like, follow, friend, or #hashtag. Yet his is a remarkable life—a story of undying commitment. It is a life defined by 1,173 incredibly consequential acts of generosity.

I am also struck now by the parallels between this story of the quest for a cure or treatment for a pernicious disease and the novel coronavirus of 2019. With both, there is loss, fear, and tragedy. But there is also dazzling science, medicine, human ingenuity, kindness, and courage. These challenges—and how we respond to them—show us how connected we all are. James's story is rich with everyday acts of kindness, meaningful encounters, and the bonds that unite us. It is about one person's ability to do good in the world. If a self-described "regular bloke" like James can make such an impact, doesn't that mean there is hope for the rest of us? James is all about the human connection, and about accepting what you can do and what you are not able to do. He is about enjoying the simple things, like paying attention to the person he's talking with, making lunch for people you care for, or just showing up.

I visited James in Australia in the summer of 2019. He could not have been nicer, humbler—and in his unique way—more inspiring. We went to the blood bank in Sydney, and I visited him at his home in Umina Beach, where I saw his stamp collection (which takes up many shelves), his pug memorabilia (many more shelves), and extensive wine and port collection. I saw his garden out back with his azaleas and bromeliads and got to spend time in the kitchen where Barb loved to cook. I met James's best friend, Joy, his daughter, Tracey, and her family, and I went with James to visit Lizzie Thynne and Robyn Barlow. Both Lizzie and Robyn shared photos, memories, recordings, news stories, journals, and more.

Talking with James about his life as a donor—as the treatment, if you will—was what made me want to understand the underlying condition. My research brought me into the fascinating history of blood as both medicine and commerce. I saw the beauty and intricate purpose of blood. I also saw the dangers in blood, and the suffering of families before there was a treatment. And it and introduced me to John Gorman and his impressive mind. As a young doctor in New York, John's quest to find a cure for Rh disease began with a profound but

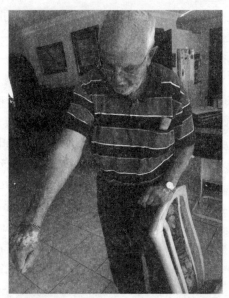

James Harrison, at home in Queensland, Australia, shows the crook of his "golden arm," where there is scar tissue after decades of blood donations.

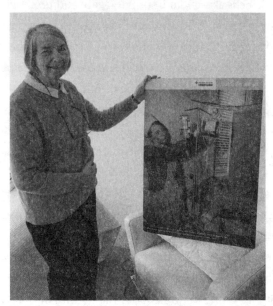

Lizzie Thynne, retired from nursing, stands next to a photo of herself in her days working for the Red Cross.

basic question: Why would a mother's body mount an immune attack against her unborn child? How could this be stopped?

John, who is not quite six years older than James, impressed me in different ways. While kind and thoughtful, he also has this "mad scientist" quality to him. Like many other successful inventors and innovators I know, he prefers looking to the future over reminiscing about the past. His ex-wife, Carol, whom I met in New York—along with his daughter Elizabeth—knows the "mad scientist" look well. As does his wife, Julia, who kept us fueled with coffee and treats during my visits to their home in Del Mar. I'm grateful to John for spending so much time with me revisiting his past and sharing the story and science of Rh. He made me appreciate a different side of medicine, one that is removed from hands-on patient care and maybe less visible. He reminded me of the behind-the-scenes work done by researchers and clinicians searching for answers and trying to move the science of medicine forward. This part of medicine is also about improving care and prolonging life.

In many respects, John and James appear to be opposites. But in reporting this multicontinental book, I was struck by the things that the two men have in common. Both are directed and disciplined. They share a love for their families. They are both ambitious, though their ambitions manifest themselves in different ways. John's ambition is about reaching goals he sets for himself—to get closer to understanding something new, to chase elusive knowledge. For his part, James's goal was simply to be the best human that he could. James always shined with his people skills, warmth and folksy humor. Over the years, as James learned the impact of his blood donations—and blood itself—he had to develop more wisdom. John's road to greatness was not just about making a medical breakthrough, but about learning to work more closely with people. In short, he had to develop more heart.

I find it interesting to think about the themes of *Good Blood*, and what the story has in common with my earlier works. Every book

I've written is an underdog story. With *The Grace of Everyday Saints*, I told the tale of a group of Catholics who fought for decades to save their historic church and waged what was the longest parish protest in Catholic America. In *The Billionaire and the Mechanic*, I wrote about Oracle titan Larry Ellison and his unlikely partnership with a radiator repairman who was head of a blue-collar boating club to go after the oldest trophy in international sports—the America's Cup. In *How to Make a Spaceship*, I wrote about Peter Diamandis's extraordinary efforts to get to space without the government's help and the brilliant and creative "outsiders" who helped him achieve his outsize dream. In *Alpha Girls*, I wrote about a group of women who succeeded in the male-dominated tech industry and helped build some of the most significant companies of our day.

Good Blood is also about going after your dreams. It is John Gorman stepping off a ship in the port of New York and setting out on a journey of discovery. It is James Harrison finding his superpower. Whether it is Gorman's brilliant mind or Harrison's big heart, *Good Blood* is about the desire to do something good and lasting in the world.

ACKNOWLEDGMENTS

A special thank-you to my talented editor, Jamison Stoltz, at Abrams, my longtime agent, Joe Veltre, at Gersh, and my friend and editor David Lewis, who has kept me sane and gotten me through every book I've written. Thank you to my family for putting up with my long hours and crazy deadlines, and especially to my son, Roman. I hope you always ask questions, look at the world with wonder, and see challenges as problems waiting to be solved.

ABOUT THE AUTHOR

Julian Guthrie is a journalist, author, keynote speaker, startup founder, and director of a national nonprofit. She spent over twenty years writing for the *San Francisco Chronicle*, where she won numerous awards and had her writing nominated multiple times for the Pulitzer Prize. *Good Blood* is her fifth nonfiction book. Her previous books are *The Grace of Everyday Saints*, *The Billionaire and the Mechanic*, *How to Make a Spaceship*, and *Alpha Girls*. She divides her time between the San Francisco Bay Area and North Idaho.

Julianguthriesf.com
Alphagirlsglobal.com

PHOTOGRAPH CREDITS

Pages 2, 24: Courtesy of the Harrison family
Page 12: Courtesy of Kathryn Gorman
Pages 16, 31, 50: By Elizabeth Wilcox, Archives & Special Collections, Columbia University Health Sciences Library
Page 25: Courtesy of the Australian Red Cross Blood Service
Pages 35, 37, 46, 231, 234: Courtesy of John Gorman
Pages 54, 136: Courtesy of Lizzie Thynne
Pages 71, 103, 128, 130: Courtesy of the Australian Red Cross
Page 109: Donor card courtesy of James Harrison
Page 151: Courtesy of Julia Gorman
Page 163: Courtesy of Val and David Semmler
Page 165: Courtesy of Tracey Mellowship
Pages 167, 170, 182, 195, 200, 219: Courtesy of James Harrison
Page 214: *Sydney Morning Herald* photograph by Steven Siewert
Page 217: Cards courtesy of James Harrison
Page 241: By the author